Healthellaneous

This Book Could Save Your Life

Dr. John Zielonka

Wasteland Press
Shelbyville, KY USA
www.wastelandpress.net

Healthellaneous:
This Book Could Save Your Life
by Dr. John Zielonka

First Printing – December 2010
ISBN: 978-1-60047-513-9

The information in this book is for educational purposes only.
All readers should consult a qualified health professional
for conditions specific to their own health.

Printed in the U.S.A.

This book is dedicated to all of my patients who have not only benefited from the health advice in my current health articles but have also entrusted me in helping them with one of their most precious assets – their health.

I would now like them to benefit from a host of new articles as well as sharing all of my articles with the rest of the world.

Table of Contents

Introduction

Over the past 20 years I have strived to not only provide my patients with the absolute best healthcare possible but to also make extraordinary efforts on educating them on what true health is all about.

I truly do believe that the word "doctor" means "teacher". Don't let anyone else ever tell you differently – you are the person most responsible for your health. Unfortunately, far too many people either expect someone else to take charge of their health, they find someone else to blame for their health or they rely on information (often from supposedly reputable sources) that is either misleading, wrong or an outright lie.

That's where I'm different. I'm going to tell you the truth regardless of how much you (or even other health professionals) may disagree. My position is quite simple – how on earth do you make an informed decision if you've never been properly informed?

Over the past few years I've had hundreds of people with the exact same misinformation and the exact same problems. After verbally repeating the same information over and over again it became apparent that thousands of others had the same incorrect information that was having significant adverse affects on their health. While you may understand how some of this misinformation came from unscrupulous marketers, much of it also came from doctors, drug companies, the government and in fact society as a whole. Hence, I began to write to inform not only my patients but also the world at large. My health articles have been discussed on television and a variety of different mediums. I have substantially added to my collection with never before seen articles that cover an incredible variety of topics including answers to the following;

1. What do scientists say is the best form of treatment for headaches?

2. Can you safely lose 23 pounds of **fat** in thirty days?

3. What is the best way to slow, prevent and reverse arthritis?

4. How can improper backpack use have your child end up in the hospital?

5. Can a blind man climb and reach the peak of Mount Everest?

6. What daily activity is the #1 cause of acute liver failure?

7. Do you really have all the facts when considering the swine flu vaccine?

8. What three things must everyone know about their spine and nervous system?

9. Why is it essential that you put yourself first?

10. What do the world's best athletes know that you don't?

11. What common problem from sitting can mimic a heart attack?

On the whole we're not even close to knowing everything there is to know about health, but at the same time we do know well more than enough to be much healthier than we currently are as a society. Please enjoy each of my health articles as well as sharing and recommending them to your family, friends and loved ones so that they may achieve the same benefits that so many have already enjoyed.

1

Taking Care of Me

Why it's essential that you put yourself first

If you're reading my articles for the first time I can understand how the title of this one could imply that I'm advocating a selfish attitude and a lack of caring for others. On the other hand, anyone who knows me would tell you that this couldn't be further from the truth.

I couldn't imagine going through life without helping others. In my professional life I'm fortunate enough to be able to use my hands and brain to get sick people healthy and keep healthy people healthy. The effort I put into educating the public about health goes well beyond my patients and well beyond most other health professionals as I truly believe the word doctor means teacher.

My personal life includes the all-important job of being there for my three children and serving as the best role model I can be. If I'm not there for them then who will be? Add a wife, siblings, friends, and helping to care for elderly parents.

Finally, I consider the charity work I do to be a privilege rather than an obligation.

And yet, as much as I care for others, if I didn't take care of myself, a lot of that care would not be possible.

Which one are you?

Are you the stereotypical mother who's had it engrained in her that it's her job to take care of everyone else first?

Are you the not as stereotypical father who acts the same way?

Or are you the friend who can never say no to others?

If you're doing any of the above, I'm here to tell you that not only should you change your ways, you **must** change your ways.

Don't I need to help others?

Of course you need to help others. As I said before, I couldn't imagine going through life without doing so nor could I imagine a world where everyone just cared for themselves. That's not what I'm advocating. Caring for and helping others is not only the right thing to do from a moral point of view, but it may also be necessary for your happiness, sense of fulfillment and overall well-being. In fact, it ironically could even be construed as meeting your selfish need to make the world a better place.

Why you must put yourself first

If you don't put yourself first, who will? It's your job and your responsibility. If you truly believe your purpose in life is to help others, how will you accomplish this if you burn yourself out? If you truly believe it's your job to take care of others, then part of that job is taking care of yourself so that you're able to complete that job. This doesn't mean that you sit on the couch for eight hours watching football while your young children go hungry but it does mean that there are times when you must put yourself first, especially in matters of your own health. Make (not find) the time to exercise, eat regular nutritious meals, take mental breaks, have social contacts and take time for yourself.

Speaking of health...

Are you someone who says that your health is your most important priority yet you spend no time achieving or maintaining that priority? Your actions must be congruent with your beliefs. If you believe that your family and your children are your most important priorities, then consider what would happen to them without your health.

Failing to ever put yourself first is likely to eventually end in burnout and ill health. It will certainly result in unhappiness and frustration. Ironically, the people that you're always putting first will perceive this and find you too irritable or unhappy to be around.

Don't sell others short – especially those you love

Did you ever consider that by doing everything for everybody you may actually be doing them a disservice? If caring for yourself is your responsibility, then caring for another is their responsibility. It's one thing to help someone – it's quite another to do everything for them. In essence, instead of helping them you may actually be re-enforcing their lack of responsibility and lack of self-esteem.

This is especially true in children. Parents often believe it's their job and responsibility to give their children a better life than they had. In many cases, however, this has gone so overboard that by doing everything for them we have actually failed to properly teach them independence and self-responsibility, making them less able to handle the real world and stand on their own two feet. This in turn may lead to a vicious cycle in which the parent feels like they have chronically failed in raising their child which leads to the need for even more care on the parent's part.

It's time to put pen to paper

Take a few minutes right now (you're entitled) and write down all the things that you do for others versus what you do for yourself. First and foremost see if there's a balance and appreciate everything you do. Then go over the list again and determine when it would be better for others that you not do everything for them and that they actually learn some responsibility on their own.

Finally, add the things that you would like to do for yourself and enlist others to help you achieve them. Not only will it be good for you but in turn it will be good for others. In fact, if it makes you happier you may find that others will be all too pleased to have a happier you. Last but not least, if you truly believe that you should help the world, why would you deny anyone else the same opportunity?

When the oxygen masks come down in an emergency situation on an airplane you are instructed that you must put your mask on first. Failure to do so could result in your death and that of your loved ones.

If you're waiting for there to be thirty-four hours in a day to take time for yourself, that's never going to happen. In fact, you'd probably take the extra ten hours each day just to do more for others. It's time to put yourself first as of right now – doctor's orders.

2

Ice or Heat?

Applying common sense to your injury

What decision could be easier? You've just injured yourself whether it be a sports injury, car accident, fall, lifting, twisting or other strain. Whether it's your back, neck, shoulder, knee or elbow, you simply decide on two completely opposite forms of early treatment, ice or heat. Then why do so many people still get it wrong?

Part of the reason is misdiagnosis and not looking at the underlying cause of the injury. The other part is rules carved in stone by some health professionals which sometimes defy common sense.

When an injury occurs the body immediately sends out an inflammatory response to the injured area, an event which is one of the very few times when the body is wrong. Usually the body has an incredible innate ability to heal itself but in this instance it treats an injury like it does an infection. This inflammatory response actually has an adverse affect on the injury and as such reducing it as soon as possible is key not only to a quicker recovery and pain reduction but also to prevent further damage.

If an area is inflamed it should be iced. What could be more straightforward? Hence, the "carved in stone" rule that you ice an injury for the first 48 hours and apply heat afterwards. Here's where the confusion begins.

**What magical event occurs at the 48-hour mark,
where at one minute before 48 hours you're icing
the area and at one minute after 48 hours
you're doing the exact opposite?**

The 48-hour "rule" is a guideline only. If you're still inflamed 96 hours post injury you should still be icing. When you do ice, apply it using the guideline of the 10-10 rule. This means 10 minutes on, 10 minutes off, 10 minutes on, 10 minutes off and so on. When you're tired of doing this, put it on for another 10 minutes. The more you can ice in the early going the better. If the body part is larger (i.e. lower back) then the time can be increased by a few minutes, if smaller (i.e. a finger) then decreased by a few minutes. Also ensure that the affected area is actually achieving the results you want. I have seen patients wrap their ice in towels so thick that the affected area is not even cool to the touch. A *thin* layer of cloth should be used solely to prevent frostbite which can occur on bare skin. Only when finished icing should you apply some Biofreeze or Deep Cold, which should be lightly applied. Repeatedly rubbing in such a gel will actually result in a heating effect.

The second confusing aspect occurs in misdiagnosing the underlying cause of the problem. We tend to live in a symptom-oriented world which means patients often judge the problem solely by their symptoms instead of what actually created the problem. Whereas a car accident or sports injury is fairly obvious, what does one do for acute low back pain? The patient will often feel muscle spasm and as such apply heat thinking that heat is for muscles. The problem is that the cause is almost always that the vertebrae or joints have become misaligned (subluxated) and the nerve is "pinched". Since the muscles attach to the vertebrae and are controlled by the nerve, the muscles tighten in response. The "pinched" nerve, however, also causes inflammation. While heating the area may originally feel nice to the muscle, you are just heating the inflammation. **You don't need to be a doctor to know that you shouldn't heat an already inflamed area.** This is typical of the person who soaks in a hot bath at night. The heat will originally feel nice as heat does ease up muscles and it will de-stress you. However, these people wake up stiff as a board the next morning and can't figure out why. They've aggravated the situation by putting heat on an inflamed area.

It can become even worse for cases of an antalgic posture where the pressure on the nerve is so great that the body's self-defense mechanism literally pulls you over to one side to take pressure off the nerve. Obviously the muscles will tighten to pull you off the nerve but again we would not apply heat to the tight muscle as this would only be a feeble attempt to overcome this self-defense mechanism. (This is why I would never recommend muscle relaxants for an antalgic posture).

If it is a muscle problem and only a muscle problem (i.e. no injury but rather a good workout) then heat is appropriate to speed lactic acid removal. With the exception of rare conditions like rheumatoid arthritis which don't really like ice, **ice is appropriate in 99% of the cases post injury.** It is almost impossible to go wrong with ice whereas heat can certainly have adverse affects.

I would also recommend a really good natural anti-inflammatory (the best on the market right now is "Acute Injury Plus" from Core Science). I much prefer the natural anti-inflammatories as not only are they effective but you also avoid the potentially serious side effects of all over-the-counter and prescription anti-inflammatories. (See my article "Anti-inflammatories – Their Side Effects Could Be More Serious Than You Realize, chapter 7).

Only when the inflammation is significantly reduced or eliminated should you then move to the ice and heat phase. Heat will serve to increase blood flow to the area and remove toxins while the ice will keep the inflammation reduced. In this instance the order of application is important where you should always end with ice to ensure the inflammation is not aggravated.

Lastly, ensure that your injury also receives the professional care it needs to address the underlying cause of the inflammation. If you are still inflamed a month or two post injury, you obviously need more than ice and natural anti-inflammatories. If a pinched nerve is creating the inflammation, you need to "un-pinch" the nerve.

Applying common sense to both your injury and overall well-being is the best way to achieve optimum health and optimum performance.

3

Headaches Are Not Due to a Lack of Tylenol

Discover the one treatment that most doctors are not aware of

One of the questions I ask all of my patients who suffer from headaches is; "What is the normal number of headaches?" The immediate response is "do you mean per week or per month?" They are surprised when I tell them that it doesn't matter what the time frame is because the normal number of headaches in a week or a month or a year is the same; zero! There is nothing "normal" about getting a headache.

Yet millions upon millions, including twenty percent of all children, suffer with headaches. Given this, you would think that modern medicine would have developed a great treatment for headaches, but the truth is that headache advice from their MD is the leading condition that patients are dissatisfied with.

What many people are surprised to learn is that doctors of chiropractic see almost as many patients for headaches as they do for low back pain and with great success. While this has been known by chiropractic patients for decades many in the medical world are not aware of this.

Dr. Peter Rothbart M.D. (a Canadian anaesthesiologist) and a team of medical researchers at the University of

Syracuse discovered almost fifteen years ago that *"Chiropractors were right. Many headaches are caused by damaged structures in the neck and scientific evidence proves it."* Your headaches could have unknowingly resulted from a fall off a swing in childhood and not manifested itself until years later.

"We couldn't believe it at first. We've been able to put together a scientific explanation for how neck structure causes headaches."

Dr. Rothbart also said that a century ago headaches were treated by drilling holes in the head and today's treatment hasn't advanced that much since that time. *"We couldn't believe it at first. We've been able to put together a scientific explanation for how neck structure causes headaches – not all headaches but a significant number of them."* He went on to say that most medical doctors are unaware of this fact.

World renown researcher Dr. Nikolai Bogduk M.D., PhD and Professor of Anatomy agrees: *"The people in control of the headache field seemingly have not, cannot, or will not, recognize this paradox; that the model for cervicogenic headache is not only the best evolved of all headaches but is testable in vivo, in patients with headache complaint. No other form of headache complaint has that facility."*

"A century ago headaches were treated by drilling holes in the head and today's treatment hasn't advanced that much since that time."

How do I know if chiropractic care can help my headaches?

Obviously you should visit a chiropractor. Your chances that your headaches are neck related are probably pretty high given that if nothing else has worked to date the neck is the likely culprit.

To know for sure, a chiropractor will be looking for any of the following; if a "pinched nerve" in the neck is the cause of your headaches a chiropractor will be able to feel this. When your chiropractor does find it you will feel tender. Further, if the nerve is pinched your neck range of motion will be limited. If your chiropractor finds any one of these three then your chances for success are good. If none of these three are present then it is unlikely that your headaches are neck related.

Advanced technology

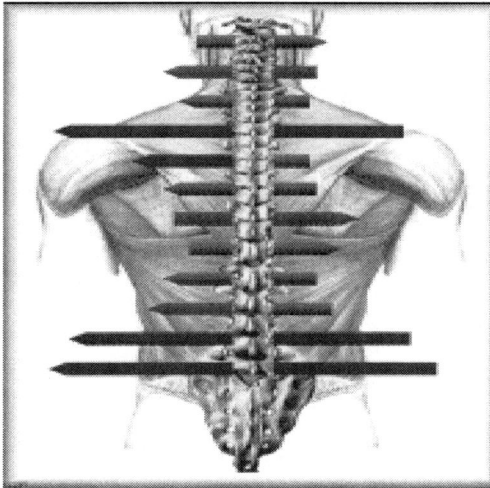

While the above three factors will be examined, a fourth factor now exists: technology. I utilize the MyoVision 8000 Nerve & Spinal Scan in my office that can actually measure the electrical activity in the neck area for any abnormalities. Lastly, any good chiropractor will attempt to rule out any "red flags" which could indicate the rare possibility that your headaches are due to an emergency situation such as a tumour, stroke or aneurysm. If you've had the same headaches for years these conditions are unlikely, simply because –to be blunt– you would have been dead long ago.

Special concern should be applied to any headache that sees a sudden unexplained change in frequency or intensity.

Chiropractic treatment

Chiropractic care's success is attributable to the fact that it actually gets to the underlying cause of the problem. Headaches are not due to a lack of Tylenol – in fact, sometimes the drugs used to mask headache pain actually cause headaches. If a nerve is "pinched" (from daily stress, poor posture, old injuries), what on earth makes more sense than to "un-pinch" the nerve?

Chiropractic adjustments are a gentle, pain-free treatment that restores the nerve and vertebrae back to normal. When done by a chiropractor, this is one of the safest and most effective forms of treatment that exists, in fact far safer than taking a single Tylenol.

"Chiropractors were right. Many headaches are caused by damaged structures in the neck and scientific evidence proves it."

Dr. Peter Rothbart MD

You have nothing to lose

Why live with something that is not normal when medical science says it is likely curable? You have nothing to lose other than your headaches and the long term side effects of the drugs you're taking to mask the pain. Remember, most MDs haven't heard of this, which probably explains why patient satisfaction with their advice is so low. Go see your family chiropractor today.

4

Take the Day Off For the Sake of Your Health and Print Your Doctor's Note While You're At It!

What all Canadians, and the rest of the world, need to know about health

If you regularly read the newspaper, (or watch television or follow the internet) you may have seen the following headline:

National Health Day

Health and Wellness Expert Declares
February 15, 2010 as National Health Day
Mayor of Ottawa Proclaims It for Nation's Capital

Six years ago I spearheaded a movement to finally accomplish what many Canadians had been asking for over the last two decades. Canadians have always prided themselves on their health care and have always wanted an extra holiday between New Year's and Easter over our long winter. Instead of waiting for the continual debate on who to name the holiday after, I simply combined the two and did something unique in government circles – I took action. Hence, we now have **National Health Day**. The Mayor of the city of Ottawa, his worship Larry O'Brien, has once again joined my quest in proclaiming National Health Day for the nation's capital as have previous mayors for the sixth year in a row.

Each year I write letters to every Member of Parliament including the Prime Minister and Minister of Health. I have made numerous television appearances including CBC and the A-Channel, as well as nation-wide newspaper and radio coverage. I wrote to Ontario Premier Dalton McGuinty almost five years ago with the idea, and while he turned me down at that time I was both surprised and pleased to see that "Family Day" suddenly appeared the very next year.

What is National Health Day all about?

It's very simple. As much as Canadians claim to be health conscious, the truth is that the majority of the public, the majority of health professionals and the vast majority of politicians don't even know what the word *health* actually means. Please appreciate that I'm not talking about serious genetic problems or severely under-privileged people who deserve much better. I'm speaking of the majority of industrialized nations who have the means and ability to be far healthier than they are. If you disagree then explain our "health care system", which is really a sick care system that attempts to manage disease. One simply needs to look at demographics to realize that such a system is doomed to failure.

There is a dictionary definition to the word health.

HEALTH *"The optimal state of physical, mental and social well-being – and not merely the absence of disease or infirmity."*

It is necessary to understand that there are three key points to this definition;

1. The definition doesn't just tell you what health is, it also tells you what health isn't. The fact that you don't have a disease or that you're not sick or not in pain does not mean that you're healthy. I know of no other word in the English language that is defined in this manner. It would be like defining an apple as a fruit that is not a banana.

2. It is a completely holistic approach (physical, mental and social well-being – I would even add spiritual).

3. By its definition health is "optimal". Therefore, there is really no such thing as being "fairly healthy" or having "average" health. In fact, even using the phrase "optimum health" is really being redundant.

Hence, on National Health Day all Canadians need to do two simple things. One, learn the actual definition of the word health and two; Canadians are encouraged to do anything healthy on this day (although they should obviously practice health every day of their lives).

I take this a step further where I actually close my office for the day and give my employees the day off with pay, encouraging others to follow suit. While some business owners will complain of the cost of a new day off, please remember that I am a business owner too. More so, this is really not about the government or employers; it's a personal decision that each person must make as they are ultimately responsible for their own health and should make it a priority for the rest of their life. Even without the day off we need to understand that our entire system still misses the mark on health and it's up to us to change that. To continue to wait for the government to take quick action on our health is really an oxymoron.

Finally, I invite the public to visit my website at www.excellenceinhealth.com to print my doctor's note encouraging that people take the day off. I would challenge all employers to be proactive and give their employees the day off with pay for the sake of their health, as a healthy workforce will provide many other benefits to employers.

If all Canadians, especially politicians and doctors understood what the word actually meant, and more importantly acted on it, our country would be a much better place.

5

Do I Really Need To Take Vitamins?
The Question Answered Once and For All

It should be easy. Either you need vitamins or you don't. Yet while billions of dollars are spent on vitamins and nutritional supplements every year, others firmly believe that they can get everything from their diet and even others believe that vitamins are nothing but "expensive urine".

These are, of course, all beliefs. But what if I told you that I could answer the question, once and for all? Not simply my opinion, but on a rational, logical flow chart approach to answering the question.

Do I need vitamins?

To answer this question, we need to know what a vitamin is and what it does. Do you? Most don't.

Vitamin – "an organic compound that can be transformed in the body into a coenzyme that aids in specific chemical reactions in the cells and tissues. Thus they are essential for physiological function"

So the answer is simple. You do need vitamins because they are essential for physiological function. But of course it isn't that easy because when we ask the question "Do we need vitamins?" what we are really asking is "Do we need them in a pill form?" So the real question is not do I need vitamins (you do) but rather...

Do I need vitamin supplementation?

I did say that it was a logical flow chart approach, so to answer this question I must, in fact, ask and answer another question:

Can I get everything I need from a balanced diet?

This can only be answered by asking:

What do I need?

This of course brings us to a key part of the question and a discussion of recommended daily allowances or RDAs versus optimum health. Is it your belief that RDAs are sufficient for health or do you strive for optimal health and what exactly is the difference? To begin to answer this, we must ask our next question:

What is an RDA?

Believe it or not, far too many people believe that these are numbers derived at some scientific high-level meeting held by the government with your best interests at heart that will give you all the health you need. The truth is that an RDA is:

RDA - "The amount of a vitamin necessary to prevent a disease deficiency."

What does that mean? It means that the RDA for vitamin C is how much vitamin C you need so that you don't get the disease that's caused by a lack of vitamin C. What disease is that? Scurvy! The RDA for vitamin D is how much vitamin D you need so that you don't get rickets! (Rickets is a significant "softening" of the bones.) This of course begs the real question:

Is this your health goal?

If your desired level of nutrition and vitamin intake (whether through diet and/or supplementation) is simply to avoid scurvy, rickets and other deficiency diseases, then meeting RDA levels would be sufficient to accomplish such a goal. Please be aware, however, that this has nothing to do with optimum health or the health continuum and is, in fact, a major contributor to why we have so many unhealthy people on this planet.

Is your health goal simply to avoid scurvy?

If your health goal is optimum health, there are thousands of scientific studies that confirm the role of supplementation in helping you achieve this and how vitamin levels well above RDA levels are necessary.

It is interesting to note that there is the occasional study that is anti-vitamin and even more interesting to note that the anti-vitamin person will rely on the one negative study to justify their position while ignoring the 100 positive ones.

Getting back to our flow chart of questions in discussing RDAs versus optimum health, one must now ask:

Can I get these (RDA or optimum health) levels from diet alone?

You would think the common sense thing to do would be to investigate this question, so that's exactly what I did. I went to Canada's Food Guide and took a **random sampling** to comprise my meals. For instance, if it said to have X servings of a food group and there were X number of pictures in the guide, I took one of each. I then calculated the actual nutrients I would get from those meals. The results?

A random selection of Canada's Food Guide for the following nutrients for the average adult:

Vitamin A   Vitamin C
Vitamin B1   Vitamin D
Vitamin B2   Vitamin E
Vitamin B3   Calcium
Vitamin B5   Magnesium
Vitamin B6   Iron
Vitamin B12   Zinc

Which ones achieved an "optimal health level"?

Not a single vitamin obtained an optimum level (as determined by a consensus of multiple scientific studies)! Hence, the answer is simple.

If your goal is to achieve optimum health and optimum levels of nutrition, you must supplement.

Please remember that the word is *supplement*, which means vitamin products **in addition to** good meals.

But what if you're really stubborn and stuck in your old sick care paradigms?

As inadequate as RDAs are, how many people actually meet RDA levels?

Youngsters' Diets Found Inadequate
~The Associated Press~

"Hold the chips and pass the broccoli! Only 1 percent of Americans ages 2 to 19 met all government guidelines for a healthy diet, a study has found."

Of course, the next question is:

Did Canada's Food Guide meet all RDA levels?

Believe it or not, our random sampling found that following Canada's Food Guide did not even meet RDA levels for vitamins E, B5 and B12.

Please note that Canada's Food Guide also did not originate at that high-level meeting with your best interests at heart. Rather, it originated during World War II as a food rationing program.

Hence, while it is a nice belief that you get everything you need from your meals, it's just not true 99.9 percent of the time. There are numerous factors that affect nutrient quality such as pollution, pesticides, soil quality, food contaminants, processing and cooking methods.

There are also factors that affect your vitamin requirements, such as physiological and psychological stress, infection, exercise, alcohol and poor nutrient density.

How many people fit into the above categories?

What about those who believe that God never intended us to take vitamin supplementation or that Mother Nature provides everything we need? I could simply tell you it's an unhealthy belief but the reason I bring it up here is that you **were** right, except you were right some 10,000 years ago. As best as can be accurately determined, it is estimated that mankind did achieve optimal levels from what we ate 10,000 years ago. So God and Mother Nature did intend us to eat healthy, we just went out of our way to screw it up.

What about the people who think that vitamin supplementation results in "expensive urine"? They're lacking the B vitamins they need for normal brain function. That's like saying that water has no purpose since it just comes out as urine. Again, it's easier for them to believe that the vitamin-takers must be wrong and wasting their money than it is for them to accept that they're not interested or willing to invest in their health.

Poor nutrition, or more precisely a lack of optimum nutrition, is involved in every degenerative disease known to mankind. Beyond helping to prevent disease, optimal nutrition is essential for optimal health. **Once and for all, do you need vitamin supplementation? The answer is absolutely yes!**

Finally, we must go one final step in realizing that not all vitamins are created equally. While this may sound very much like a cliché, you do get what you pay for. That doesn't mean that all expensive vitamins are good, it just simply means that most cheap ones, including some very well known brand names, aren't. Different vitamins are made from different sources with different binders and fillers. Most well known drug store brands have very poor absorption and dissolution. Paying less for a vitamin which is only absorbed three to five percent is not a bargain. Make the investment and buy your vitamins from health professionals that you trust.

Do I need vitamins?

↓

Do I need vitamin supplementation?

↓

Can I get everything I need from a balanced diet?

↓

What do I need?

↓

RDAs or Optimal Health. What's your goal?

↓

Can I get this from my diet?

↓

Almost always, NO.

↓

Once and for all, do you need vitamin supplementation?

↓

The answer is absolutely YES!

6

Are You In the Minority?

The number of people receiving alternative health care may surprise you

"Humans were designed to be healthy as long as they are whole. Body, mind and spirit. People are characterized by self-healing properties that come from within and an innate healing force. Perfect health, harmony is the normal state for all life."

The above sounds very much like a cross between the actual definition of health and chiropractic care. Or, if you are a staunch medicine-only supporter, you might say some alternative or natural health gobbledegook. But the truth is that the above is a quote from Hippocrates some two thousand years ago. For those of you who don't know, Hippocrates is widely recognized as the father of medicine.

I find it hard to believe that I've been treating patients for over twenty years now yet I still remember when I first started. It was not uncommon back then to have patients insist that I not tell their medical doctors that they were seeing a chiropractor. While I'm pleased to say that this has changed significantly over the past twenty years (I regularly get medical referrals, have medical doctors, surgeons and chiefs of staff as patients, and was even asked to be present when an MD was giving birth to provide care to her newborn baby) there still exists the rare misinformed MD who is anti-alternative health.

What do the actual numbers tell us?

Harvard Medical School conducted a study back in 1991 (nineteen years ago) that found that the number of visits to alternative health care providers actually exceeded the number of visits to medical doctors by thirty-seven million visits in a single year in the United States. A follow-up study was conducted in 1997 (six years later) that found while the number of visits to MDs decreased by two million visits, the number of visits to alternative healthcare providers actually increased by over two hundred million visits. As such, those patients who were reluctant to tell their MDs or friends that they were receiving chiropractic or some other form of alternative health care, feeling that they were in the minority, were actually in the majority and have been for at least the past twenty years. Put another way, if you're not receiving some form of alternative healthcare you're actually in the minority.

The World Health Organization estimates that 65 to 80% of the world's population relies on alternative healthcare as their primary form of healthcare.

Why is that?

While governments and drug companies have done their best to mislead you, the truth is that healthcare, like everything else, is in the hands of the consumer. People have begun to realize that their health is their responsibility and that they're willing to pay for it out of their own pocket. Consumers spend billions out of their own pockets (non-insurance coverage) on alternative healthcare in a single year (2 billion on vitamins alone in Canada and 22.5 billion on vitamins in the US). While many people have private insurance to help with these costs, most such plans are sorely lacking or limited and many other people have no such coverage at all. It is also rare that anyone has coverage for vitamins, yet many have rightly concluded that not only are you allowed to spend a dollar of your own money on your health but in fact what better investment could you make? Health care does have a cost but it usually pales in comparison to the cost of not having your health.

Who leads the alternative healthcare movement?

Of all visits to alternative healthcare providers, sixty-five percent of those visits were to chiropractors. Chiropractic easily forms the largest form of natural health care in both Canada and the US. In fact, many chiropractors even dislike the use of the term "alternative" health care. There really is no "alternative" to taking care of your spine and nervous system as chiropractic care does. Please appreciate that medicine manages disease. Chiropractic (and most natural healthcare) provides health. Again, is the "alternative" to providing health not providing health? How is it that the father of medicine's quote sounds so much like health and chiropractic and so unlike what we know medicine to be today?

The bottom line

If you've been receiving chiropractic and other forms of natural health care for some time now – congratulations! Chances are you're much healthier because of it. If you haven't, why are you and your medical doctors still in the minority? You and your health deserve better.

"Humans were designed to be healthy as long as they are whole. Body, mind and spirit. People are characterized by self-healing properties that come from within and an innate healing force. Perfect health, harmony is the normal state for all life."

Hippocrates

7

Anti-inflammatories -
Their Side-Effects Could Be
More Serious Than You Think

If you think that people are insane when it comes to nutrition, they're even more insane when it comes to drugs. Consider this;

You're in pain. It could be low back pain, a headache, a fall, sports injury, car accident or even your arthritis. And you do what millions of Canadians and Americans do every day. You reach for a pill. You're looking for the quick fix and what's wrong with just a pill or two, especially if it's going to make you feel better? After all, if millions are doing it and they're all approved by the FDA and Health Canada, what could possibly go wrong? The truth? The truth is that plenty could go wrong. And not just to the rare person but to thousands. Let's look at the facts, but first a little background.

Three types of drugs - Drugs for pain basically fall into three different categories: pain killers, muscle relaxants and anti-inflammatories.

- **Pain killers** – These include common over the counter drugs such as Tylenol. Why am I generally anti-Tylenol? Because it does absolutely nothing to fix the underlying cause of the problem and simply masks the pain. Why is masking the pain a problem?

Because pain is your body's warning system that something is wrong. By masking the pain not only are you short-circuiting this system, you may actually go out and aggravate your condition even more. Not to be blunt, but no one ever died from pain. Furthermore, they do have their side-effects, especially so in children as much as we feel the need to do something for our kids. I only recommend pain killers in cases where they would allow for sleep which is necessary for proper recovery and health.

- **Muscle relaxants** – As much as I don't like pain killers, I like muscle relaxants such as Robaxacet even less. Again, think *underlying cause*. People want quick fixes and think symptoms. In most cases the muscle is not the underlying cause but rather has reacted to the irritated nerve or dysfunctional joint. This is especially true in seriously impinged nerves that result in an antalgic posture where the body's self-defense mechanism is literally pulling you off to one side off the nerve. Why would you want to try to defeat the body's self-defense mechanism and put pressure right back on the nerve?

- **Anti-inflammatories** – This is the one type of drug that makes sense as we do want to bring down inflammation as quickly as possible. Inflammation after an injury is one of the rare times when the body's innate wisdom messes up. It treats injury the same way it does infection and long term inflammation is actually adverse to our health. This is why we should ice an injury immediately. Anti-inflammatories include over the counter drugs such as Advil, Ibuprofen and Motrin as well as prescription drugs such as Naprosyn, Voltaren, Arthrotec and Celebrex. So what's the problem with anti-inflammatories? There are many.

The side effects of anti-inflammatories

While you may believe that drugs are "safe" because they've been approved by Health Canada or the FDA, you'd have to be living under a rock not to be aware of the multiple drug recalls from supposedly "safe and approved" drugs. It is fairly common knowledge that anti-inflammatories can be tough on your stomach but do you know to what extent? Last year, 76,000 people went to hospital emergency rooms in the U.S. due to the "side-effects" of anti-inflammatories, many suffering from serious stomach bleeding and even death. Last year in Canada alone, 1900 Canadians **died** from anti-inflammatory use.

The new death rate

Think it can't happen to you? We all know that studies can contradict one another. However, a few years ago, two scientists looked at every study that had ever been completed on the "chronic" use of anti-inflammatories and came up with a new **death rate**. How did they define "chronic"? Chronic was defined as anyone who had been using anti-inflammatories for two months or longer. This would include anyone with chronic headaches, arthritis, menstrual problems, chronic injuries and so much more. Please note that anti-inflammatories were only ever meant to be used in the short term meaning two weeks or less. If you still have inflammation two months later, obviously you're not correcting the underlying cause of the problem.

So what was the death rate? What are your chances of dying from taking anti-inflammatories for two months or longer? Is it one in a million? One in a hundred thousand? The new death rate is **1 in 1,200**. (This is not a misprint.)

The natural alternative

Aside from using ice, (chapter 2 "Ice or Heat? ~ Applying common sense to your injury") there are many natural alternatives that are not only effective but extremely safe. My highest recommendation goes to Core Science's Acute Injury Plus. Based on the latest science and research, not only is it highly effective and of unparalleled quality, but it even has components which double as a digestive aid. Hence, instead of harming the stomach, it actually benefits the stomach. For best results it should be taken immediately after discovering the inflammation and continued until the inflammation is gone, while also addressing the underlying cause of the injury.

8

Subluxated Ribs May Mimic a Heart Attack

You're experiencing a sharp pain and tightness in your chest. It hurts to take a deep breath in. It might be accompanied by anxiety, worry or stress and maybe even neck, shoulder or arm pain. It's even worse if there's a history of heart disease in you or your family. Do you call 911? Do you rush off to the hospital emergency department to spend hours waiting? Or do you ignore it?

Needless to say, ignoring such symptoms is never a good idea. It is possible that you're actually having a heart attack and given the potential consequences, no matter how small the risk, this must be properly examined by the appropriate health professional without delay.

But what happens after all the waiting, after the examination and ECG and after all the additional stress created by the thought that you were having a heart attack when your medical doctor tells you you're "normal" and they can't find anything wrong?

It could very well be a subluxated rib.

What is a rib subluxation?

If I were to ask you to point to your ribs you'd probably put your hands just above your waist in the front – and you'd be right. But you actually have twelve pairs of ribs which extend all the way up to the base of your neck and wrap all the way around in the back attaching to your spine. This essentially forms a suit of armour to protect your heart and other vital organs.

A subluxation is the scientific term used by chiropractors that usually refers to spinal vertebrae which have become misaligned and are thus interfering with normal nervous system flow. These subluxations (not dislocation) come from daily stressors which can be physical (chronic work posture, poor posture, injury, imbalances), chemical or emotional.

Therefore; a rib subluxation is a misalignment of a rib. The most common are your third, fourth or fifth ribs which, because they wrap around over your chest and heart, may create chest pain or muscle tightness mimicking a heart attack. They may also be felt in the upper back just inside your shoulder blade. Finally, since your ribs expand and contract with each breath, if they are subluxated (think jammed or stuck) it may be difficult or painful to take a deep breath in.

How are these fixed?

Contrary to the MD who said you were "normal" or that nothing was wrong, a rib subluxation is not normal and must be corrected. To be fair, the MD was far more concerned that you weren't about to die from a heart attack but to also be fair and accurate, many MDs have never heard of a rib subluxation and certainly don't know how to fix it. (In twenty years of practice I've had one MD recognize this and refer the patient to me.)

The best and really only way to fix such a subluxation is through chiropractic adjustments. If your rib is jammed and pinched, what on earth makes more sense than to un-jam or un-pinch it? The good news is that a chiropractic adjustment is a very safe and effective way to correct this rib dysfunction. The bad news is that rib adjustments are notorious for being difficult adjustments "to hold" as most people unknowingly have significant weakness in their postural muscles surrounding this area, especially if they sit at a desk for a living. As such, a series of chiropractic adjustments are necessary. This, combined with the appropriate spinal stabilization exercises and proper ergonomic advice has a very high rate of success even for chronic conditions.

In some cases relief may be almost instantaneous but again, full correction, followed by stabilization, is mandatory as many people go right back out into the real world which created the problem in the first place. The worst case I have ever treated was a patient who swore that he was having a heart attack so he spent hours in emergency. The hospital, after examination and even performing an ECG, couldn't find anything wrong with him so they sent him home with both Demerol and Percocet – not just one narcotic but two. Five days later he still had his heart attack pain and finally came in to see me. (He should have known better since he was a patient of mine.) Five minutes after I adjusted him his heart attack pain was gone.

A colleague of mine experienced a different twist treating a patient in Saskatchewan. My colleague used to see quite a few farmers who were familiar with rib subluxations due to the nature of their work. As such, many farmers would automatically go straight to their chiropractor, recognizing that it was a rib subluxation and not a heart attack. In this one case, however, the farmer came in to my colleague saying "doc, it's that rib again but this time it's different – I have significant numbness down the left arm". Needless to say, my colleague sent the farmer straight to the emergency ward.

In closing. . .

Again, many MDs are unfamiliar with this as it simply isn't their specialty or area of expertise. This, combined with the added anxiety and lack of effective treatment after a heart attack has been ruled out, can be both painful and frustrating. If you're experiencing this and you're sure it's not a heart attack, it's time to see your chiropractor.

9

Are You Walking Around in Circles?

The truth about leg length discrepancies

One of the most misunderstood aspects of posture and proper pelvic alignment is the concept of having your legs being of different lengths.

I have had patients who believe that everyone has different leg lengths (or that all chiropractors tell you so) and I have seen x-rays taken by one of the best hospitals in Canada showing that if your pelvis is not level then you must have two different leg lengths. Both of these beliefs are wrong.

What exactly is a leg length discrepancy?

Quite simply a person lies down on their stomach with their legs straight and one looks at the bottom of their heels to determine whether their legs are of equal length.

Why is this important?

Put this same person into an upright standing position and consider all the effects such a leg length discrepancy would have. A leg length discrepancy of even ¼ or ½ an inch would cause significant postural changes. Your pelvis, hip and shoulders would all be un-level. More body weight would be carried on one side. Every step (the average active person takes ten thousand in a day) would result in more pressure leading to everything from plantar fasciitis to increased wear and tear and resulting degeneration. This degeneration would not be limited to the foot but would also affect the ankle, knee, hip and in fact the entire spine. Muscle imbalances would be present which would certainly affect athletic performance. Overall energy levels would even be affected as the body would be forced to deal with the extra strain. Even your overall height could be decreased.

This of course would affect nervous system function and hence anything in your body could be affected. Lastly, bear in mind that just a ¼ inch is considered significant from a biomechanical point of view. While this is common there is absolutely nothing normal about this. As a runner picture if your leg had to go an extra ½ inch on one side with every step just to hit the ground.

There are two different types

The key thing to understand is that there are two different types of leg length discrepancies.

A **true leg length discrepancy** is one in which if I were to pull both your legs off and actually measure them they would be of different lengths. This can also be measured with a tape measure while your legs are still attached to you by utilizing what are known as the appropriate landmarks. It is rare that people have a true leg length discrepancy. It occurs in people with rare genetic conditions or those who have actually broken their leg in the past.

An **apparent leg length discrepancy** accounts for more than 99% of all leg length discrepancies and while common, is definitely not normal. It occurs when the pelvis (especially the sacroiliac joints) become subluxated or misaligned through chronic work postures, muscle imbalances, poor posture, stress, injury and lack of proper spinal maintenance. Since the legs attach to the pelvis, any misalignment in a forward or upward direction will pull the leg with it giving the appearance of a leg length discrepancy with all its adverse effects as previously mentioned. (This is why a pelvic x-ray in no way confirms a true leg length discrepancy.)

How does one fix this?

The best treatment by far (and usually the only treatment) is chiropractic care. If the leg length discrepancy is an apparent one as the result of pelvic or sacroiliac misalignment, then what on earth makes more sense than to correct this subluxation by realigning the pelvis? The results of chiropractic care can sometimes be dramatic and immediate where even one adjustment can often show a change in leg lengths. In fact, if I have another family member in the room when I adjust a patient I will often show them the immediate post treatment effects. (Without that family member some patients find such an immediate change almost unbelievable.)

That's the good news. The bad news is that it is unlikely to stay that way after just one adjustment as the body has become used to the misalignment as well as its accompanying weaknesses and imbalances. However, with a series of adjustments combined with the appropriate stabilizing exercises (both are necessary) my clinical experience has shown a 99% success rate in correcting this dysfunction.

How should you not treat this?

With a heel lift as some health professionals wrongly advise. Why? Because while you may think that you're equalling the difference in leg lengths, you're doing so by ensuring that the pelvis stays permanently misaligned. The only time that a heel lift is appropriate is for the rare apparent leg length discrepancy that fails to respond to chiropractic care or for the rare true leg length discrepancy.

**99% of all leg length discrepancies
are apparent leg length discrepancies.**

Apply the above common sense solution to your leg length discrepancy and not only will you reap the health benefits, you'll also stop walking around in circles. See your chiropractor today.

10

Your Painkiller May Be Killing More Than Just Your Pain

What Tylenol doesn't want you to know

The last time I checked one of the goals of medicine and the government's role in our so-called healthcare system was to help eliminate as many causes of disease and dysfunction as possible. In fact, the well-known adage "first do no harm" is widely considered as one of the fundamental principles of medicine.

As such, imagine if we could eliminate some of the causes of heart disease, diabetes, arthritis and cancer. Needless to say it would be difficult to disagree with doing so and immediate action would be taken.

What about acute liver failure? What if I told you that it's in our power right now to immediately eliminate the number one cause of acute liver failure in the U.S? Would it not be our duty to do so immediately? Of course it would be.

What is the number one cause?

So just what is the number one cause of acute liver failure? Let's be clear. Not one of the causes but **the** number one cause. Is it alcohol abuse? Is it viral hepatitis? No, the number one cause of acute liver failure is the consumption of acetaminophen, the main ingredient in painkillers such as Tylenol.

When acetaminophen is ingested there is a rapid depletion of glutathione in the liver. Glutathione depletion results in the free radical destruction of liver cells.

Just how bad is the problem?

In the U.S, acetaminophen poisoning results in 100,000 calls to poison control centres, 56,000 emergency room visits, 26,000 hospitalizations and more than 450 deaths from liver failure.

Regular acetaminophen users may also double their risk of kidney cancer. Last, but certainly not least, the excessive free radical formation can cause damage throughout the body and has been implicated in most major diseases, especially those which are age related.

Acetaminophen use is the number one cause of acute liver failure and doubles your risk of kidney cancer.

But don't I need to take my Tylenol?

Why? Tylenol is a painkiller. I know that's an obvious statement but a painkiller does nothing to fix the actual underlying cause of the problem, it simply masks the pain. Excuse me for being blunt but no one ever died from pain. In fact, it's your body's warning system to tell you that something's wrong so that you'll take the appropriate action – not short circuit your warning system.

Furthermore, masking the pain may allow you to engage in activities that unknowingly create even more damage or delay proper treatment. From a marketing point of view however, it's exactly this strategy that allows drug makers to create lifetime patients and make billions of dollars in profits.

A drug company would never put profits ahead of our health would they?

Yes, of course I realize what a naïve question that is, but let me give you some specific examples that you may not be aware of;

- Infants were ending up in hospital emergency wards with acute liver dysfunction when it was discovered that infant strength Tylenol was actually significantly stronger than children's strength Tylenol (as opposed to the other way around)

- A lawsuit revealed internal memos from Tylenol that instructed its sales reps not to discuss the adverse effects of mixing Tylenol and alcohol. While you may consider it common sense not to mix drugs and alcohol, the memos apparently revealed Tylenol's knowledge that adverse effects could occur from taking Tylenol many hours after alcohol consumption. What do thousands and thousands take for their hangover?

- After the above issues were revealed, Tylenol continued to market itself as the "safest" pain reliever on the market. I still remember watching the spokesperson on television whose response to the above was simply how anti-inflammatories were even worse. Scary, isn't it?

So what do you do?

If we truly lived in a rational world we would immediately eliminate the gross overuse of acetaminophen and thus eliminate the number one cause of acute liver failure. We would also cut the risk of kidney cancer in half and lessen the risk of most major diseases simply by stopping the taking of just one drug.

The bad news is that we don't live in a rational world. The good news is that you get to choose. I can't remember the last time I took a Tylenol (and that's not due to memory loss). We're not talking years but rather it's been decades since I last took a Tylenol or other acetaminophen product.

Stop relying on painkillers. Realize that their adverse effects are far more significant than you realize and that if you're taking them they are having an effect on you – not just on the other guy. Consider natural alternatives, fix the actual underlying cause of your pain if possible and seek professional advice from qualified health professionals. Better yet, practise a lifetime of health so that most chronic conditions never occur in the first place.

11

Metabolic Detoxification & Intestinal Cleansing - How to Clean Yourself From the Inside Out

My late favourite aunt was a nutritionist extraordinaire, who always used to say that if she could do only one thing to improve a person's health it would be to turn them inside out and brush them off. She was absolutely right. Proper nutrition is one of the 5 Keys to Health, of which metabolic detoxification and intestinal cleansing is a key component.

Think of your body like a blast furnace. On a daily basis you consume a number of different foods and substances voluntarily as well as a number of other substances involuntarily. Now consider that these substances contain pesticides, pollutants, toxins, second hand smoke, chemicals, preservatives, drugs, antibiotics, carcinogens, poor quality nutrients and a number of other undesirable components. No matter how hard you try (assuming that you do) what will the inside of your blast furnace look like over time? Now consider that this same blast furnace, essentially covered in years of "crusty black soot", is still responsible for effectively absorbing the proper nutrients and excreting the toxins from your body. It is little wonder then that this malfunctioning system can lead to fatigue, headaches, lack of mental clarity, bloating, weight gain, digestive troubles, irritable bowel, muscle and joint pain and a variety of significant diseases. This dysfunction occurs whether you feel its effects or not as your body's systems are over-stressed and forced to work overtime with less than optimal results. Times have changed in this over-polluted world. This is why regardless of your beliefs, a proper detox program is essential for everyone who desires optimum health.

A proper detox program

Not surprisingly, there are many different products of varying quality on the market. A proper program requires each of the following components:

1. **The proper nutrients**
   A proper detox program appreciates that you have likely caused damage to your system. Hence, specific nutrients are necessary to repair this damage. As such, a proper detox program will contain the "**4 Rs**";
   a) **Repair** – Specific nutrients are needed to repair the damage that you have done to your intestinal lining. This prevents the proper nutrients from escaping where they shouldn't, as well as allowing for the toxins to be excreted where they should.
   b) **Remove** - Other specific nutrients are then needed to kill off the bad bacteria.
   c) **Replace** – Good bacteria and other probiotics must be added to your system to allow for proper function.
   d) **Rejuvenate** – The liver must then be detoxified, which again requires specific nutrients to help restore it to normal function.

2. **The right foods**
   During your detox program, your health professional should provide you with a list of specific foods you should eat as well as those to avoid. Quite simply, you do not want to eat the

same toxin-filled foods while trying to detoxify. This can lead to the introduction of new healthier foods as well as being able to go on a counter rotation diet after your detox which will often allow you to identify foods that you may crave but are actually bad for you.

3. **Proper supervision**
   While benefits may certainly be seen from doing such a program on your own, a proper detox program is best when under the supervision of a qualified health professional that can anticipate and be prepared for how your body may react. Will a "die off" period occur (where your symptoms may originally increase as toxins exit the body)? Will there be some interaction with any prescription drugs that you are taking? (Always consult your medical doctor if this is the case.) What should you do if bloating occurs? These are all questions that a qualified health professional can answer.

Just who is a qualified health professional?

Anyone who has advanced nutritional training. This may include your chiropractor, naturopath, homeopath, advanced nutritionist and maybe your dietician, nurse or medical doctor. Please note, however, that many MDs and some dieticians may not necessarily get much training in advanced nutrition and in fact many "health consultants" may sometimes understand this topic much better.

Can't I just fast?

In a word, no. While many people fast for religious reasons, this is the equivalent of putting less in the blast furnace. Weight loss may occur and you may be giving your system "a rest" but you will never achieve proper detoxification and repair as this requires very specific nutrients.

What are the best detox programs?

In my office I utilize three different programs depending on the patient's needs and their health goals. The programs are provided by different labs, all of which are considered to be the best in the world. The majority of these programs are not available in nutrition stores or drug stores so that they may be properly supervised with professional support.

i)   **Comprehensive Detox Cleansing Program -** This program typically lasts three to four weeks (longer for cases of fibromyalgia and other serious conditions) and may cost in the $300 to $500 range. Suppliers may include Douglas Laboratories or the Ultra Clear program. While this may initially seem expensive it will replace some meals which some people break down to $5 to $10 per meal. Also consider its value. It is a small price to pay for a properly functioning liver and digestive system.

ii) **Starter Detox Program -** This type of program lasts seven to ten days and costs in the $150 to $250 range. Suppliers include Core Science, Douglas Labs and Isagenix.

iii) **Easy Man's Detox -** Don't let the name fool you. While the other two programs are more comprehensive, this super convenient program from Core Science or Douglas Labs in the $75 to $100 range has significant benefits.

The best programs (as described above) are backed by decades of well researched scientific evidence versus what you are likely to find in a drug store or on the internet. Given that new research shows that years of poor nutrition is just as bad for the liver as years of alcohol abuse, it is all the more essential that you consult a qualified health professional. They can also guide you during the process and properly instruct you about things such as a "die off" period where you may actually see symptoms increase as toxins escape.

Who Should Detox and When?

Again, everyone should detox and in fact given today's society should do so on a regular basis. I personally detox three to four times per year to help ensure that my liver and intestinal system function at an optimal level year round. Some of my patients find that timing is the bigger problem where they don't want to detoxify around holidays, birthdays, vacations, social events and travel. Unfortunately, it is exactly this lifestyle that results in your current less-than-optimal status. A good detox program is not hard but does require some discipline. The benefits, however, can be amazing. This may include increased energy, fat loss, better mental clarity and concentration, better organ function, less bloating and much better overall health.

12

Time Doesn't Heal Everything

One of the biggest misconceptions people tend to have is that time heals everything. This may or may not be true in love, relationships and past experiences but that's not my area of expertise and hence I won't comment as to its validity.

When it comes to "time heals all wounds", again this could be referring to love and relationships or may be taken literally in reference to health. This simply isn't true. Let me give you two scenarios.

Scenario #1

You bend over to pick up something and out of the blue you experience a sharp pain in the lower back with a pins and needles sensation referring into your left buttock. In addition, you experience significant muscle spasm which pulls your body over to the right and alters normal walking as well as affecting your sleep.

You're concerned enough that you make your way immediately to your medical doctor's office and after waiting two hours (six hours if it's the hospital) she examines you. After a number of tests she tells you that she's concerned but is not going to give you any treatment. Instead, she wants to monitor the situation closely where she instructs you to come back and see her again in two weeks. She also states if the pain's too bad you can take Tylenol.

Scenario #2

The exact same injury occurs but instead of going to your MD you tell your story to the guy working at the counter in the Mac's Milk store. He tells you to do nothing and hopefully it will go away in two weeks. He also tells you if the pain's too bad the Tylenol is in aisle 3.

What's the difference between scenario #1 and scenario #2? Absolutely nothing other than scenario #2 saved you two to six hours of your time. If you think I'm kidding look at the end result. Your MD may have been very well meaning but unless you're the rare case whose back pain is coming from an underlying tumour or aneurysm that just happened to be brought on at the exact same moment that you were picking up something, in both cases nothing was done. There was no treatment, no discovering the actual underlying cause of the problem and no difference in the final prognosis. Both the MD and the Mac's Milk guy are hoping the problem will go away with time.

(The correct answer, of course, would be scenario #3 in which case you would see your chiropractor.)

This "do nothing approach" is based on the belief that many injuries are what are referred to as "self-limiting". Self-limiting is the belief that a majority of injuries require no treatment and will simply get better with time. The reason this belief is dangerous involves a number of factors;

1) Just because the pain goes away doesn't mean the problem and its underlying cause have been corrected.

2) Getting the appropriate treatment can speed recovery and lessen pain faster.

3) Doing nothing may in fact simply delay appropriate treatment which allows the condition to become chronic. Conditions which have been neglected and

allowed to become chronic require significantly more treatment to correct.

4) While the percentage of cases which become chronic may be small, chronic conditions (in the case of low back pain for instance) account for ninety-six percent of the cost of treatment.

5) Conditions which have been allowed to become chronic or where treatment has been delayed actually speed up the advancement of spinal degeneration.

As such, waiting for time to heal things is never a good idea. Please appreciate that chiropractors are bigger believers than anyone in the body's incredible innate ability to heal itself but that only occurs when the body is working properly.

A broken arm takes six weeks to heal but only with proper treatment (i.e. a cast). Try going six weeks without the cast and see how well your arm heals.

It is not time that heals everything, rather, doing the appropriate things over that time. Following the same logic, age doesn't create health problems, rather it's what you do or don't do as you age.

Unfortunately, most people believe in wishful thinking and are looking for excuses to absolve themselves of their self-responsibility. Why take a logical, rational and comprehensive approach to health when you can rationalize your lack of time, inconvenience, lack of priorities and lack of effort? Waiting for something to go away is no different than waiting for it to come back.

The most common words heard in a chiropractic office – "I thought it would go away."

Remember that in cases such as our scenario, most injuries are insidious in nature. That means that everyday stressors such as chronic work posture, postural imbalances, mental stress and chemical exposure have been building on a daily basis long before you feel any effects. Only seven percent of the nervous system even perceives pain, and symptoms are the last thing to appear just as the arteries of your heart begin to clog up long before your heart attack.

This is actually one of the things for which chiropractic doesn't get enough credit. If you break your arm and your MD puts a cast on it you don't go home and bang your arm against the wall a thousand times. If your dentist puts braces on your teeth you don't go home, pull out a pair of pliers and start fiddling with the wires. In chiropractic, what we spend a few minutes correcting, you then spend the rest of the day doing the exact same things that threw your spine and nervous system out of whack in the first place. (This explains the need for regular care especially in the early going instead of time in between care.)

Take the appropriate action today.

If time cured everything then everyone would actually get better with age. Stop looking for the quick fix and stop hoping that doing nothing is your best course of action. Take the appropriate action so that you can maximize recovery, not minimize treatment and effort.

**It is not time that heals everything, rather,
doing the appropriate things over that time.**

13

What Do the World's Best Athletes Know That You Don't?

Have you ever heard of Tiger Woods? How about Lance Armstrong? Don't forget Wayne Gretzky and Michael Jordan. Now add Joe Montana, Jerry Rice, Dan O'Brien, Evander Holyfield and yes, even Arnold Schwarzenegger. Last, but certainly not least, Muhammad Ali.

What do these people have in common? Many things. First and foremost, they are some of the best athletes the world has ever seen. Aside from being incredibly gifted, their dedication, work ethic, perseverance and effort is outstanding. They never solely relied on their God given talents (Michael Jordan was actually cut from his high school basketball team) but rather did everything they could to achieve peak performance in their sport.

What else do they have in common that allowed them to achieve and maintain their peak performance? They are all staunch supporters of regular chiropractic care.

Tiger Woods, arguably the best golfer in the world prior to his recent troubles, has been quoted as saying that his chiropractic care is as important to him as practising his swing. Lance Armstrong, arguably the best athlete of all time actually takes his chiropractor on tour with him and has said that there is no way he would have won seven Tour de Frances without chiropractic. Wayne Gretzky and Michael

Jordan used chiropractic to help them become the best players in their respective sports.

What about Joe Montana and Jerry Rice? Jerry Rice, one of the greatest wide receivers to ever play in the NFL is actually a spokesperson for chiropractic. Joe Montana, holder of four Super Bowl rings and three Super Bowl MVPs is also the spokesperson for chiropractic in the state of California. You may in fact recall being one of hundreds of millions who saw Joe Montana (and 35 team mates) receive chiropractic care during a special segment on national television just prior to the start of the 1990 Super Bowl.

Dan O'Brien, former decathlon gold medalist has stated "If it were not for chiropractic, I would not have won the gold medal". He went on to say:

"You obviously can't compete at your fullest if you're not in alignment. And your body can't heal if your back is not in alignment. It was the holistic idea that I liked about chiropractic and that is what track and field is about. Every track and field athlete that I have ever met has seen a chiropractor at one time or another. In track and field, it is absolutely essential. Chiropractic care is one of the things I think that no one has denied or refuted."

Dan O'Brien

What about boxers Muhammad Ali and Evander Holyfield? Muhammad Ali's performance clearly transcended beyond sports. As for Evander Holyfield;

"I have to have an adjustment before I go into the ring. I do believe in chiropractic. I found that going to a chiropractor three times a week helps my performance. The majority of boxers go to get that edge."

Evander Holyfield

What about Arnold Schwarzenegger? While you may think of him as the Governor of California or the action movie star, don't forget that he got his start as the athlete who revolutionized body building.

"Bodybuilders and fitness people have been using chiropractic very extensively in order to stay healthy and fit. I found it was better to go to a chiropractor before you get injured. We are a perfect team – the world of fitness and the world of chiropractors. That's why I always will be traveling around, all over the world, talking highly about the profession of chiropractic. You chiropractic doctors are really miracle workers."

Arnold Schwarzenegger

What does this have to do with me?

It has everything to do with you.

First, if chiropractic can help the world's best athletes (and this is only a very small sampling) achieve peak performance, imagine what it can do for you in your everyday life.

Second, people sometimes get the mistaken idea that exercise can replace chiropractic. This couldn't be further from the truth. It's a safe bet that the athletes mentioned here all exercise more than you or I do. Exercise doesn't reduce the need for chiropractic, rather it increases it. Exercising on a spine that's subluxated or misaligned actually increases your potential for injury and leads to an increase in degeneration.

Third, chiropractic care maintains spinal alignment, optimizes nervous system function, improves balance, power, strength, flexibility, stability and peak performance. While excellent for injury recovery, maintaining your spine and nervous system at an optimal level can actually prevent many injuries from ever occurring in the first place.

The world's best athletes receive regular chiropractic care not only for injuries but to achieve and maintain peak performance

Your beliefs are impacting your health

If you still believe that you can achieve peak performance in your sport or everyday life without chiropractic, you're quite simply wrong. If that were true, then you must be more successful and know something that the world's best athletes don't. And while you may believe that a belief can't be right or wrong, it can certainly have an impact on your health.

"I found it was better to go to a chiropractor before you get injured"

Arnold Schwarzenegger

14

Start the Year Healthy

How to help ensure your New Year's resolutions result in a year of energy, peak performance and optimum health

You're likely to be one of those many people exercising in the gym in January. The bigger question is whether or not you'll still be there in February. Unfortunately, many people often think of their health only twice a year: New Year's day and on their birthday. New Year's resolutions can in fact be a very healthy practice, if they are used properly. Are you taking stock of your current situation, setting very specific achievable goals and have an action plan to achieve them? Or are you setting the exact same resolutions that you have for the past ten years having never achieved them? If so, it's time for a different plan.

New Year's resolutions date back to early Roman times around 153 BC. Breaking New Year's resolutions is almost as old.

For some, setting a plan for January 1st is just a way of procrastinating in November. There's nothing magical about January 1st that couldn't have started November 17th or December 9th. Here are some simple strategies that you can use to help ensure you follow through on your goals and make this your best year yet.

Setting goals

Take an hour to sit down and set some specific goals IN WRITING. Decide what it is that you really want AND are prepared to make the effort to accomplish. If you're simply looking to break one bad habit, that shouldn't take long to do. If you're looking for an overall change in your existence the plan could be quite comprehensive.

Your resolutions and goals must be SPECIFIC. To simply say I want to "get healthy" doesn't mean much. There are five Keys to Health which go well beyond just nutrition and exercise. Are you looking for regular exercise, quality nutrition, daily vitamin supplementation, a good detox and cleansing program, quality sleep, regular spinal health, daily relaxation and healthy beliefs? Will your exercise be strength training, cardiovascular, stretching, core strength or rehabilitation? Are you looking for strength, endurance, fat loss, flexibility or injury prevention? Are you more concerned with an arbitrary number (lose ten pounds or take an inch off your waist) or would you like to increase your energy, feel better and be able to do the things you want? As you can see the plan can become quite comprehensive.

Make it realistic

If you get winded simply walking up one set of stairs and haven't exercised in a year, the new master plan of working out seven days a week may be doomed to failure. If you hate running and are a late riser, the newly planned 6am run in winter weather may not be your best choice. Ideally you should choose activities that you enjoy. If a chronic injury has been hampering your activities, it's time to get it fixed once and for all.

If there's a particular food that you love, never eating it again is unlikely to work. Instead, choose to eat it once a week. There is compromise between every day and never.

The best time of day to plan

While everyone talks about how the morning is the key to your day, the best time of day to plan is the night before. Take five minutes to plan your meals for tomorrow. Do you have the food? Is your lunch packed? Do you have food for dinner? Have you run out of your vitamins? Is your chiropractic appointment booked? When are you meeting your personal trainer? Is it time to see your massage therapist? Are your gym clothes packed at the door? Don't let the morning rush be an excuse to not achieve your goals.

Enlist the help of others

I strongly believe in the old Chinese proverb that I'd rather teach you how to fish than feed you every day. Having said that, I also appreciate that even the best athletes in the world (who likely exercise more than you and I) all utilize personal trainers, even though they are fully versed on exercise. Do you have a good nutritionist, a good chiropractor, a good massage therapist and more? Professional help and motivation can be key to helping you accomplish your goals and stay on track. Enlisting the help of others can also include non-professionals. Tell your friends, your family and even enlist "health partners" as one more way of making you accountable to your goals.

Adaptability

The word "decide" literally means that you have "cut off all other possibilities". Hence, if we have decided to get healthy we simply do. However, in the real world we are faced with many obstacles on a daily basis where our health goals often lose their priority. Your plan must be adaptable and there must always be options. If you missed your morning vitamins take them at dinner, don't simply skip them until tomorrow. If an emergency came up that caused you to miss your afternoon workout, make it up in the evening. If you're traveling, push-ups and sit-ups can be done anywhere. There can always be an excuse to skip something. You want to achieve your goals, not have a list of excuses no matter how valid you think they are. It is said that new habits can be developed in as little as two weeks. The problem is that your old habits were practised much longer than that. It will always be easy to go back to your old ways. Remember, you're not looking for easy.

You want to achieve your goals, not have a list of excuses no matter how valid you think they are.

What do you do if by January 9th you've already fallen off your program or haven't even started it yet? Begin January 10$^{th.}$ Or as Nike says, "Just Do It". Remember, the smallest deed is better than the greatest intention. Review your plan regularly, reward yourself each step of the way and make your goals a priority.

Energy, vitality and peak performance

You should think of New Year's as one more added incentive to begin a lifetime of health. Except this time you have truly decided and there is no turning back. This time, ensure you take all the steps to make it happen and experience life as it was meant to be. You deserve it.

15

Spinal Degeneration is NOT Inevitable

What you can do today to prevent your spine from aging

"You're getting older – what did you expect?" is the common response given by many doctors to explain the degeneration of your spine as you age. The problem is that this belief is a self-fulfilling prophecy as it absolves self-responsibility and results in inaction, allowing your spine to continue to degenerate.

If age were the sole factor in the degeneration of your spine, then please explain why some sixty year-olds have no degeneration while some thirty year-olds have advanced spinal degeneration. Or better yet, explain why your L_5 vertebrae is degenerating while your L_3 isn't – they're obviously both the same age. It's not age or time that causes degeneration – it's what we do (or don't do) over that time. It may be common to degenerate over time, but there's nothing normal about it.

Spinal Degeneration = Spinal Deterioration = Spinal Decay = Degenerative Joint Disease = Degenerative Disc Disease = Osteoarthritis

The most common arthritis

There are over 100 different types of arthritis, of which osteoarthritis (OA) is the most common. Contrary to common belief OA is due to lifestyle factors and **not** genetics (unlike rheumatoid arthritis). It is essentially a "wear and tear" of the discs and the joints. There are two factors which cause this degeneration:

1) **Damage**
   Quite simply, if you damage something, it will "wear and tear" faster. If your car gets in an accident, guess which part of your car will rust first? This damage can be what I call "fast damage" or "slow damage". Fast damage would include things such as car accidents (whiplash) or other types of injuries. Slow damage would include a much smaller amount of pressure but over a prolonged period of time. This would include chronic work posture, poor posture or uncorrected spinal subluxations (spinal misalignments).

2) **Lack of movement**
   I'm sure you've heard the old adage "if you don't use it, you lose it". The reason it applies here is that while most of the body receives its nutrients via the blood stream, there are no blood vessels that go directly into the disc. Hence, a disc receives its nutrients through a process called imbibition, which means the more movement **specific** to each individual disc, the more nutrients that will be pumped into that disc. A lack of nutrients would obviously be likely to result in more degeneration.

Phase 1   Thinning of the disc and/or a loss of the normal spinal curve.

Phase 2   Advanced degeneration – significant thinning of the disc and/or bone spurs (osteophytes).

Phase 3   Severe degeneration – large bone spurs and/or partial or total fusion.

The natural approach

It is important to appreciate that spinal degeneration is an ***ongoing process***, not a static condition. In other words, if you do nothing to change your ways, it is likely to progress. To have a normal spine (and not a common one), steps must be taken to a) undo the damage, b) increase spinal range of motion and c) restock the disc with the proper nutrients. This would include;

1) **Chiropractic adjustments**
   Chiropractic is an ideal form of treatment for spinal degeneration (osteoarthritis) as it can help undo fast damage, re-align slow damage and increase range of motion specific to the individual joint. (Simple stretching cannot replace chiropractic as it cannot "unlock" or realign a subluxated vertebrae.)

2) **Spinal stabilization exercises**
   This does not mean bigger pecs, biceps or running. In fact, running on a misaligned spine (just like driving your car on misaligned wheels) is likely to increase its wear and tear. Rather, these exercises must be prescribed by someone who has seen your x-rays and are specific to stabilizing the core muscles and ligaments that support your spine as well as helping to restore your normal curve.

3) **Specific nutritional supplementation**
   The nutrients (and amounts) necessary to help you rebuild your discs cannot be achieved through diet. By supplying the proper nutrients (combined with chiropractic to help ensure they enter the disc) degeneration can be slowed, stopped and in some cases even reversed. The scientific research shows that glucoseamine, chondroitin sulphate and MSN have shown positive benefits to the spine. Other nutrients such as shark cartilage, sea cucumber and bromelain-papain have also shown positive benefits.

My highest recommendation goes to Core Science's Arthri-Joint Max as it includes all of the above.

How long should it take?

Most people have unknowingly spent years allowing their spine to degenerate when in fact they should spend a lifetime keeping it healthy. Spinal correction (chiropractic), spinal stabilization and nutritional support for a degenerated spine requires a minimum of a year (and often more) for maximum improvement, just like a dentist putting braces on your teeth. Remember, you're not looking to mask the pain but rather help restore and rebuild your spine. By taking a comprehensive natural approach and addressing all three factors, your spine can last a lifetime.

16

Are You Cracking Your Own Back or Neck? Think Again!

Why trying to adjust your own spine is never a good idea.

Admit it. You probably know someone who either does this or has had it done to them. It may be "helpful" Uncle Bob who, when you mention your mid-back pain, squeezes you in a massive bear hug until you hear "crack, crack, crack" up and down your entire spine. "Doesn't that feel better?" he says. It may even be you who grabs your own neck giving it a quick jerk until you hear a pop thinking you've done a good thing. This is never a good idea. Here's why;

Subluxation and nervous system dysfunction

When you "crack" your own back, what you believe you're addressing is referred to in scientific terms as a vertebral subluxation. A subluxation is a misalignment and dysfunction of the vertebrae that results in interference and/or dysfunction of normal nervous system flow. Subluxations occur from daily stressors. These stressors may be physical (chronic work posture, poor posture, spinal weakness, accidents) emotional or chemical in nature. Since your brain is constantly sending messages to every cell, tissue and organ in your body via your nervous system, any blockages or interference has the capability of adversely affecting anything in your body.

Then what's wrong with correcting this?

There's nothing wrong with correcting this. To the contrary, it's essential that you correct it otherwise you're adversely affecting your overall health, your body's life centre is compromised, its communication system is dysfunctional and your body's innate ability to automatically repair and regulate itself is diminished long before you feel any effects. This is what doctors of chiropractic detect and correct and is essential to good health. The difference is a chiropractor is the expert at doing this – you're not.

In simple terms

To simplify this explanation, let's say that you took the nervous system out of chiropractic (which you really can't do because chiropractic is all about your nervous system).

Again, really oversimplifying, let's talk only of the joints in your spine where each of the vertebrae meets one another. They can either be normal, too tight or too loose. Obviously we want them to be normal. When a chiropractor adjusts you. . .

Vertebral subluxation
- "the scientific term for misalignment and/or improper function of the spinal vertebrae resulting in nerve interference"

Chiropractic adjustment
- "a highly skilled, highly specific, very gentle, very safe procedure performed using the chiropractor's hands to begin to correct subluxations thus realigning the spine, restoring normal nervous system function and thus allowing the body to use its innate healing abilities"

...he or she is essentially taking the vertebrae that are too tight and restoring them back to normal. Chiropractors correctly use the term "adjustment" as it is a far higher skilled and highly specific procedure versus spinal manipulation utilized by some physiotherapists and a handful of medical doctors. Whereas non-chiropractors may attempt to learn spinal manipulation in weeks or months, doctors of chiropractic spend years in honing their skills in performing chiropractic adjustments and still realize that it may take further years of practice to become really proficient. Never come to me to perform surgery; never see anyone other than a chiropractor to adjust your spine. When you (or Uncle Bob) do this to yourself, there is no way in the world that you are adjusting the vertebra that needs it and certainly not in the direction or degree necessary. (Trying to locate a subluxation solely by pain is a huge mistake.) Hence, you're not adjusting the vertebra that needs correction. (Does Uncle Bob say "yes- it's your T4 which is subluxated in 30 degrees right lateral flexion, 40 degrees left rotation and 70% extension?) Rather, when you "adjust" yourself you are moving the vertebra which is the easiest one to go – the one that is actually too loose.

Another problem. . .

This misguided behaviour is perpetuated by the fact that even when you adjust a vertebrae that is too loose you can still get what is referred to as a reflex muscle reaction which can actually ease up the muscle and make you feel better. The problem is that the loose joint gets looser and looser eventually becoming hyper mobile which can then lead to instability.

Obviously you don't want unstable vertebrae. At the same time, the joints that really need to be properly adjusted actually get tighter and tighter which may speed up degeneration in these vertebrae.

When I first met my wife she could "crack" her neck all the time. Now she couldn't do it if her life depended on it as

I've adjusted the tight vertebrae and taught her how to strengthen the loose ones.

The "crack" you may hear is not a cracking of the bones or the bone popping back in place – rather it is a release of gas (mostly carbon dioxide and nitrogen) from the synovial capsule of the joint.

The moral of the story

There is still the rare misinformed individual or even health professional who speaks out against the significant benefits of chiropractic adjustments. If they truly believe that, it is the height of hypocrisy that they have no problem with other health professionals who have a far lesser degree of skill and education performing spinal manipulation. It is even more insane that anyone would ever do this to themselves.

Chiropractic adjustments are an essential part of everyone's health care to maintain a lifetime of optimal spinal and nervous system health. In the hands of a good chiropractor, an adjustment to any part of the spine is one of the safest, most effective forms of treatment available today. Yet with all this skill, I don't know of a single good chiropractor who would ever think of adjusting themselves. Given this, why on earth would you? Even chiropractors have their own chiropractors.

17

Swine Flu
Is the Fear All Hogwash?

Two new things everyone should know

Unless you've been living in Antarctica for the past few months, it would be impossible not to be aware of all the newspaper and TV reports regarding the swine flu. Are we prepared, will it kill thousands or is it all just fear mongering?

I'll get to answer that question in just a minute, but first I would really like people to know two very key elements that are missing from all the discussion.

1. Why should we wash our hands?

Every newspaper report, health report and TV commercial has stressed the importance of hand washing and quite frankly, they are right. However, the point that is missing is asking the question of why should we wash our hands? Now again, that may seem obvious to you but understanding the answer is of key importance. Obviously we should wash our hands to prevent the spread of this disease. However, we need to understand how this disease is actually spread. It is only when the virus enters our body that it has the potential to manifest itself and result in the disease. This does not occur through the skin of your hands; rather this occurs when our hands touch any opening on our face. This can be as simple as you biting your fingernail, scratching your ear, rubbing your eyes or touching an apple and then eating the apple. When it comes to children this of course becomes much worse because they have a habit of sticking their fingers in numerous different places. Hence, what we really should be told is that we should wash our hands prior to touching our face, or more importantly that we should quite simply stop touching our face as much. This is also why we should be taught to sneeze into our elbow and not our hands.

To illustrate its importance you could have one person who washes their hands thirty times a day yet fails to do so after shaking someone's hand and then scratching their eye. They would be at greater risk for contracting the disease than someone who only washes their hands three times a day but always does so immediately prior to meals and never touches their face. While this may seem like a simple point, understanding it can make a major difference in the fight against swine flu.

2. The most important factor

The second important component that is not being discussed is actually the most important factor. While health officials are talking of preventing the spread of the flu and who should be vaccinated, the most important factor in not getting the flu is not who is spreading it to you, but rather how strong your system is to deal with it. Please appreciate that the spread of the flu is based on something called the germ theory, which was originally developed by Louis Pasteur. What many doctors and health officials don't realize is that on his deathbed Pasteur recanted the germ theory as the sole most important factor in catching a disease. If the most important factor was that someone spread it to you then every doctor, every nurse and every hospital worker would always be sick because they are always exposed to germs.

In fact, we are all exposed to germs on a regular basis.

Now you may say "Isn't strengthening the immune system done best with the new vaccine"? In a word, no. There are many other ways to strengthen your immune system on a daily basis that do not require the latest, untested vaccine. Good nutrition, adequate sleep, stress reduction, exercise and specific vitamin supplementation are all excellent ways to boost your immune system. In fact, there are many vitamin supplements specific to boosting your immunity.

Chiropractic care

What many doctors don't realize is that the largest form of natural health care in the world is also one of the best ways to boost your immune system. At last count there were well over 100 scientific studies that confirmed the role of chiropractic in boosting your immune system. One of the best-known studies involved Dr. Ronald Pero, Ph.D., chief of cancer prevention and professor of medicine at New York University. He found that patients who received regular chiropractic care had a 200% stronger immune system than those patients who didn't, and a 400% stronger immune system than his cancer patients. He also found that this increased immunity did not decline with age provided that the patient maintained their chiropractic care. This is easy for any chiropractor to understand as we realize that the nervous system controls the components of the immune system and by maximizing their function we increase our own immune competence.

Should you get vaccinated?

Quite simply this is a personal decision on your part. However, before you decide, you should be well informed and not solely from fear mongering or scare tactics. Rather, make a reasonable decision based on your health choices. There is no denying that some people have died from the swine flu but to put it into perspective, far more die on a regular basis from the everyday flu. If the vaccine was proven effective and could guarantee our safety without any risk the answer would be easy. Unfortunately, the effectiveness of the vaccine has not been proven and there is simply no time for any long term safety studies to be completed (this is true of most vaccines). In fact, to illustrate how much vaccination is based on faith rather than science, the Centre for Disease Control in Canada just released findings that show anyone who received the "regular" flu shot last year is twice as likely to catch the swine flu as those who were not vaccinated. Based on the latest reports, over fifty percent of health-care workers and other health professionals have chosen not to receive the vaccine even prior to this finding. What does this say about its effectiveness or safety?

Could it also be that they are concerned that the new vaccine contains thimerosol, a mercury based component that has been removed from most vaccines in Canada due to its association with autism and other conditions? While proponents of the vaccine may suggest that any link to autism has not been proven, neither has the effectiveness of the vaccine been proven. You can't have it both ways.

Is it cold and flu season? No, it's autumn

In the end, we all want the same goal - what's best for our health. Shouldn't that include both proof that the vaccine is 100% effective and 100% safe, especially when there are so many other safer and more natural ways to ensure our health?

18

Swine Flu - Part 2

Ten questions that we need answered

If you feel as I do then you would agree that there's been way too much reporting of the H1N1 virus. If that's true you could also ask the obvious question – why am I writing about it again? I've actually tried very hard not to write about it. In fact, according to my licensing board I'm not even supposed to have a professional opinion. For the record I'm required to inform you that 1) immunization/vaccination is outside the scope of practice of chiropractic and that chiropractors do not have the legislative authority to immunize/vaccinate patients and 2) patients should consult with health providers who have immunization/vaccination within their scope of practice (namely physicians, nurses and nurse practitioners). My licensing board is right. This is absolutely not a chiropractic issue.

Having said that I must also tell you that I've had more patients ask me and be confused about H1N1 than any other health matter in my eighteen years of practice. Without giving you a résumé, I do the most extensive community service lecture series of any doctor in Canada that I know of (55 different health lectures), I founded National Health Day in Canada, I've written numerous health articles, made dozens of television appearances and have just completed my third book "Nutrition Insanity". The point is that I'm not on a vaccination crusade but I most certainly am and always have been on an **informed decision** crusade when it comes to health. This is certainly one topic where many people are not being properly informed. Quite simply, how can one make informed decisions about their health if they're not truly informed?

What does truly informed mean?

1. It means that we are given **all** the information on a topic, both pro and con, from a reliable source that we can trust.
2. It means that the information is based on rational thought – not emotion, scare tactics or fear mongering.
3. It means that scientific facts are presented – not opinions, beliefs or dogma that is misrepresented as scientific fact no matter how long you've believed them to be true.
4. It means that we shouldn't be reluctant or fearful to question anything about our health. In fact, it is our responsibility to educate ourselves and question both our healthcare and our healthcare providers.

Who are Dr. Holtorf, Dr. Blaylock, Dr. Palevsky, Dr. Mercola and Dr. Schabas?

There is this belief amongst pro-vaccination people that anyone who is anti-vaccination must be getting their information from unreliable internet sources. In fact, if you go to the Canadian Pediatric Society's website it will even tell you how to spot an unreliable website. According to them, one such way is that an anti-vaccine website only links to other anti-vaccine websites. Apparently this same pro-vaccination site doesn't see the hypocrisy in only linking to other pro-vaccination sites. Contrary to their belief, there are many well respected experts with a different point of view.

Dr. Holtorf is an infectious disease expert who appeared on CNN in early October 2009. He stated that if he had to choose between getting the swine flu or the seasonal flu, he would prefer the swine flu. He also stated that he had more concerns about the vaccine than he did the flu, as the vaccine was shown to cause autism in children with mitochondrial dysfunction and parents would have no way of knowing if their children had mitochondrial dysfunction. When asked if he would give the H1N1 vaccine to his kids he said he definitely would not as the vaccine was a proven neurotoxin that had twenty-five thousand times the mercury that would be considered toxic in food.

Dr. Blaylock is a board certified neurosurgeon who states that H1N1 has resulted in far fewer deaths in the U.S. than that of the regular seasonal flu (900 for H1N1 vs. 36,000 for the regular seasonal flu). The same is true in Canada. He points to an investigative report done by television network CBS that contrary to the Canadian belief that if you have the flu it must be H1N1, the Centre for Disease Control apparently tried to hide the fact that its testing showed H1N1 only accounted for two percent of flu-like symptoms in states such as California and Georgia, and he believes that this is the reason they stopped testing. Dr. Blaylock goes on to point out that when the U.S. began giving flu vaccinations to children in 2003 the death rate increased seven hundred percent. He also questions why we're not following the lead of Australia and New Zealand (given their different seasons they've already had their "flu season"), which found that pregnant women are actually at very low risk (contrary to what we've been told) and that giving the vaccine to pregnant women actually resulted in increased health risks for their children.

Dr. Palevsky is a board certified pediatrician from New York School of Medicine. He states that again, contrary to popular belief, proper studies have never been done to show the effectiveness of vaccination, that they have not been proven safe, that the concept of "herd immunity" is unscientific, and that there is a big difference between developing a natural immunity from disease and what happens from vaccination. (Vaccination results in a humoral mediated response but not a cell mediated response – naturally acquiring a disease results in both.)

Dr. Mercola is a world renowned naturopath who owns what is easily the largest natural health website in the world (www.mercola.com). He states that while most of the children who died from H1N1 had an underlying chronic health condition, **all** of them had a co-occurring bacterial infection which could be a possible factor as to why "healthy" people died from the flu. He also quotes studies from the medical journal The Lancet, that giving your child Tylenol with the flu shot (likely for most parents either for fever or pain) could actually make things worse.

Dr. Schabas is a chief medical officer in Eastern Ontario and the former chief medical officer for all of Ontario. He states "To be honest I was never entirely convinced people should have been vaccinated in the first place given that the risk was so small". He also believes that the idea of a third wave is "nonsense" and is in fact being used as a convenient excuse by health officials as to why far less people have died than expected.

How can this be in such stark contrast to what we've been told?

You were taught that the theory of vaccination is pretty simple. Basically you inject a "controlled" amount of the disease into your body which then develops an anti-body and supposedly protects you, hence being given credit for having saved millions and eradicating disease.

If that's true, how is it that I can quote an infectious disease expert, neurosurgeon, pediatrician, naturopath and medical doctor who don't necessarily agree? Simple. They're brave enough to take an in-depth look at the rational science regardless of how many people believe otherwise. I say brave because it's not necessarily a great career move to be anti-vaccination on such an emotional issue. Unfortunately, most doctors don't realize what they've been taught comes largely from the drug companies.

Why did H1N1 become such a big issue?

Was it the media? Was it the drug companies? Was it the medical profession? Was it the government? Was it society's beliefs? Or was it because it killed a small number of people who were supposedly otherwise healthy which could simply mean that we haven't figured out the reason why yet?

Didn't kids die from H1N1?

Yes. And that's a tragedy that I couldn't even begin to imagine. You should also know that some children have suffered serious reactions to the vaccine. Isn't that all the more reason to ensure that we take the best rational approach to help prevent any more future deaths and future adverse reactions to the vaccine? That's why you may have heard my response to Randall Moore's commentary on CHEZ 106.1 in Ottawa, that our health decisions must be truly well informed.

Then what do we do?

We do exactly as I did when all three of my children had the flu and the same you would do for any other flu. (No, I didn't "catch it" from my children contrary to the germ theory). Watch them closely, give them plenty of fluids, ensure they get plenty of rest, watch their breathing, take good natural supplementation, minimize any drugs unless they have a high fever (there are other options) and get individual professional advice when necessary. Also, keep their immune system as strong as possible to avoid or minimize the risk in the first place. What we don't do is allow government authorities to warn and threaten to fine or jail people such as well known U.S. health expert Dr. Andrew Weil for recommending natural alternatives. Contrary to the pro-vaccine establishment, natural health professionals are not looking to make big profits from their recommendations. We're looking to give good quality expert advice to people who need it. Again, the accusation seems hypocritical given the billions that drug makers are making from the vaccine. Besides, how could anyone possibly be against people naturally boosting their immune system?

Let's be honest and reasonable with the facts

If the Ottawa Sun wants to have a section entitled "Ask the Expert" which asked why fifty percent of health professionals were choosing not to be vaccinated, then they should have actually answered the question.

If newspapers are going to report that the adjuvant is a booster that only contains fish oil, vitamin E and water (pretty healthy things the last time I checked), then they should explain why recipients of the shot are asked if they are allergic to mercury or formaldehyde.

If health officials are going to claim that they're "stumped" at some people's reluctance to get vaccinated then they shouldn't give them conflicting information that "stumps" them in the first place.

If they are going to perpetuate this long standing myth about herd immunity (see Dr. Palevsky) and claim that 80% of the population needs to be immunized, then they should explain how that will ever be achieved if only fifty percent plan to be vaccinated.

If you're telling people that children are dying from the flu then don't be surprised that they're not willing to respect the priority groups. After all, **if** you believe in vaccination and that H1N1 will kill your child, what could possibly be more of a priority?

As of the date of this article there have been four H1N1 related deaths in the Ottawa area and nine serious adverse reactions to the vaccine. Since the spring, Canada has seen 198 H1N1 related deaths (mostly with underlying health conditions) and 36 serious reactions to the vaccine that have been reported, including one death. (It still hasn't been qualified what "related" means for those dying of the flu or the vaccine.) GlaxoKlineSmith, the sole maker of the vaccine in Canada, warns that up to 1 in 1,000 people who receive the vaccine can experience an allergic reaction that can lead to a "dangerous decrease in blood pressure". Hence, if everyone in Canada was vaccinated even the drug maker expects that up to 33,000 Canadians could suffer this dangerous decrease in blood pressure.

Ten questions that we need answered

1. When the flu season is over a month or two from now will we claim that the vaccine program was responsible for keeping the death rate so low, or will we realize that just as many people didn't even get vaccinated and hence the vaccine couldn't have been responsible? On the other hand, if there is a major pandemic was it that enough people didn't get vaccinated or did the vaccine fail?

2. If the vaccine was so important how will we justify the fact that so many people saw H1N1 come and go before the vaccine was ever available to them?

3. Who is conducting a scientifically sound, quality study to demonstrate the difference between H1N1 vaccinated and non-vaccinated people? If no one is – why not?

4. If, as Dr. Palevsky concurs, there have never been any quality studies showing the scientific long term benefits of vaccination contrary to most people's beliefs, when will the multi-billion dollar earning drug companies conduct these? If not, why are we not outraged at this given that these substances are being injected into our children?

5. How will we justify it if long term side effects from the vaccine become apparent? The standard line "the benefits outweigh the risks" is unfairly touted as even the FDA reports that vaccine side effects are **ten times under-reported**.

6. Every flu strain mutates, which makes the vaccine ineffective. This has already happened with H1N1. Why has no one questioned this?

7. Will future investigation be done to determine if there is a link between H1N1 deaths and a co-occurring bacterial infection to explain why "healthy" people died?

8. It was believed we had to do something. Was this belief correct and did we do the right thing?

9. Will this approach of having a vaccine for everything (drug companies are now working on a vaccine for smoking and obesity) have the same long term effect as the overuse of antibiotics?

10. Will this approach eventually result in people questioning all vaccinations?

In closing

I never have and never will tell a patient whether they should or shouldn't get vaccinated. I will, however, tell them that they should be truly informed (since often they only hear one side of the story – in this case paid for by your tax dollars) and then make the best health decision that they can for them and their family without fear or emotion. (For every child you show me that suffered serious consequences from a disease that you believe could have been prevented with a vaccination I can show you a child who suffered serious consequences from the vaccination.)

I will also tell all levels of government that Canadians deserve an honest answer to all of the above questions. When you can answer the above questions to your satisfaction, make your decision and then relax knowing that you've made the best decision that you could based on all the facts. After all, we all want what's best for our health and our children.

19

Eight Year-Old Lifts 18 Tons

Parents often underestimate the importance of backpack safety

Fact #1

Depending on which year, over the past decade anywhere between **5,000 and 12,000** children visit hospital emergency rooms in the U.S. each year due to injuries from backpacks.

Fact #2

Studies in Canada, the U.S. and even New Zealand show seventy-five percent of children will experience a musculo-skeletal injury. This means there is only a twenty-five percent chance that your child won't.

Fact #3

There has been a thirty percent increase in back pain in children since 1990 – largely attributed to backpacks.

Fact #4

A twenty pound backpack lifted on and off just five times in a day equals ten lifts. Ten lifts times twenty pounds equals two hundred pounds a day. Multiply this by one hundred and eighty school days in a year and your eight year-old has just lifted **thirty-six thousand** pounds or eighteen tons in one year!

While some parents are beginning to realize the importance of backpack safety, many still don't realize that it is imperative that they invest the time to ensure that their children's backpacks are safe and appropriate. Ill fitting backpacks result in back pain, neck pain, headaches and shoulder pain not just now but in the future. As a result both decreased activity and energy levels may be present. Prolonged use leads to postural changes, altered gait, spinal damage and even nerve damage. It may also aggravate scoliosis, especially prevalent in teenage girls. The high number of emergency room visits is also due to a significant increase in falls from heavy or unbalanced packs, including tripping over them or falling down stairs. Remember that many of these childhood problems turn into chronic conditions in adults. Most importantly, remember that all this is happening to a growing spine.

How much should my backpack weigh?

A backpack for high school students should weigh no more than fifteen percent of their body weight and a maximum of ten percent for elementary students. This means your fifty pound eight year-old's backpack should weigh no more than five pounds while a fifteen year-old who weighs one hundred and twenty pounds should carry a maximum of eighteen pounds.

What should parents and kids look for in a backpack?

- Proper size – bigger is not always better. The top of your backpack should be no higher than your shoulders and the bottom no lower than your waist.
- Choose canvas or vinyl over leather as it is lighter.
- Wide padded adjustable shoulder pads are a must.
- A hip or waist strap is essential to keep the weight close to your body.
- Individualized compartments help balance the weight.
- Built in back supports or even wheels may be a consideration.

How should it be worn?

- Always over both shoulders. Hanging a backpack over one shoulder will cause significant imbalance and future problems.
- Straps should be snug but not too tight.
- Close to the body with the heaviest objects closest to the body.
- Evenly distributed.
- Watch out for pointy objects.
- Don't take what you don't need.

When putting it on or taking it off use both hands, bend at the knees, lift with your legs and ideally place the pack on a desk or have a friend help you.

Prevention is key

The above will work only if it is practiced. Talk to your child about proper use and its importance. In addition, good posture and core strength is invaluable. Lastly, spinal check-ups are essential to ensure proper alignment before you ever put your backpack on your spine. You would never think of not taking your child for an eye exam or dental exam, why on earth would you not take them for a spinal exam by your family chiropractor?

Remember that those eighteen tons are in a single year. Carrying that backpack for fifteen years is **two hundred and seventy tons,** and that's just the time lifting it, not the time carrying it. It's little wonder then that seventy-five percent of kids suffer a musculo-skeletal problem. Don't roll the dice – beat the odds by following all of the above for backpack safety and the health of your child.

20

Motor Vehicle Accidents & Whiplash

What you can easily do to lessen the damage and even help prevent them in the first place

Staying off the road would work. Or better yet, just have everyone else stay off the road. Of course, I assume you were looking for a more practical answer. The truth is that most (if not all) motor vehicle accidents are avoidable through better driving, cars in good working order and driving suitable for the road conditions. Unfortunately, we all know that doesn't always happen.

There are two additional simple and effective things that everyone should do to lessen the damage from a whiplash injury and in fact even avoid an accident in the first place.

1. Proper headrest placement

This literally takes ten seconds to do yet you would be surprised at the number of people whose injuries are actually made worse by the improper use of their headrest. A whiplash injury is referred to as a hyper- flexion hyperextension injury. This is because upon impact the head is thrown violently forward and then violently backward. Proper positioning of your headrest will prevent the hyperextension component thus resulting in less stress and strain to the nerves, joints, muscles and ligaments. Most people's headrests are too low, simply sitting at the lowest position on the top of their car seat. Not only does this not prevent the backward movement, it often results in what is known as a "ramping" movement. When this happens the headrest actually serves as a fulcrum which results in an exaggerated backward movement and more damage.

Take ten seconds now to ensure
that your headrest is properly adjusted

Proper headrest placement is such that your headrest is approximately midway between the top of your neck and top of your head with the head being no more than one to two inches in front of the headrest.

2. Preventing car accidents in the first place

While many people know of chiropractic's success in treating whiplash (as well as many other injuries resulting from a car accident), what if I were to tell you that chiropractic care could actually prevent a car accident from happening in the first place? Let me explain.

Many car accidents occur because people don't, or can't, properly check their blind spot. Unless you've had this checked by your chiropractor or other qualified health professional who has quantitatively measured you, most people don't realize that they have lost their normal neck range of motion. Chiropractic is highly successful at improving and correcting this lack of normal movement which comes as a result of everyday stress, chronic work posture, previous injuries, degeneration and people's failure to adequately maintain their spine. Stretching alone rarely works. As such, regular chiropractic care would actually result in fewer injuries (and fewer deaths) in the first place.

Two true patient examples come to mind. The first was a patient of mine, whom upon measuring her neck range of motion I asked her if she found it more difficult to check her blind spot. Her response was: "Are you kidding, how do you think I got in an accident in the first place?" The second patient was even scarier. She came in one day repeatedly thanking me. When I asked her what she was thanking me for, she described how she was driving along, was going to change lanes, checked her blind spot and saw a big truck, so she obviously didn't change lanes. Again I asked her what she was thanking me for and she responded: "Well, before you had fixed my neck I would have changed lanes anyway."

Are you one of these people and don't realize it? You should be able to turn your neck, both right and left, such that your nose is directly over the mid-point of your shoulder. Most people unknowingly cheat where it is their eye looking over their shoulder and cheat even more so because their shoulder is hunched forward. A clear sign is when you instinctively turn your shoulders to make up for what your neck can't do.

If you are in a car accident

Just as everyone should have regular chiropractic care in the first place to maintain their spine and help prevent car accidents, did you know that chiropractic care is one of the best forms of treatment for injuries sustained in a car accident? **Did you further know that under Ontario law you are fully covered for all reasonable and necessary chiropractic care to return you to your pre-accident state?** Think about it. In a whiplash injury the typical approach is a neck brace and pain killers. If the nerves are pinched, the joints are jammed and the muscles are stressed, wouldn't it make more sense to gently and effectively "un-pinch" the nerves, "un-jam" the joints and ease the muscles followed later by specific stabilizing and strengthening exercises?

Who should get checked?

Absolutely everyone should get properly examined by a spinal expert after any motor vehicle accident no matter how minor you think it was. A quick response is essential to a quicker recovery and to avoid future problems. Furthermore, symptoms often do not appear until days, weeks or even sometimes months later. In these cases, the pain is then often not attributed to the accident but rather longer work hours or increased stress. Most importantly, whiplash and other car accident injuries (especially if not properly treated or if proper treatment is delayed) may lead to increased spinal degeneration which is wrongly attributed simply to aging. (Please see my article on spinal degeneration, chapter 15)

The Moral of the Story

- Take ten seconds right now to properly position not only your headrest but those of all of your passengers.

- Have your neck range of motion checked and corrected by your chiropractor, especially if you failed our simple tests.

- If God forbid you are in a car accident, not only should you be fully covered for the cost of all reasonable and necessary chiropractic care (without any need for a medical referral) but you will also find it extremely safe and effective.

By following the above, our roads and more importantly the health of you and your loved ones, will be better for all.

21

Three Things Everyone Needs to Know About Their Nervous System and Spinal Health

There are three essential common sense concepts that everyone needs to understand and apply to their spine and nervous system.

1.   Everyone needs a chiropractor for life

Regardless of your beliefs, you still have a spine and nervous system. While you may never have been taught this, they are of vital importance to your overall health. Chiropractors are doctors who are spine and nervous system specialists. Could you *"get by"* without ever seeing a doctor of chiropractic? That all depends on how you define *"get by"*. You can also *"get by"* without ever exercising, with eating junk food, with little sleep and with a poor attitude. Just don't expect to be healthy. Your spine is like anything else. Anything you don't maintain will eventually create a problem. Imagine if you never brushed your teeth. You wouldn't be surprised when they started to fall out. Your spine houses your nervous system which is the master controller of everything that goes on in your body and controls every cell, every tissue and every organ. Unfortunately, we are all subjected to stressors such as chronic work posture, emotional stress, old injuries and postural imbalances which adversely affect the integrity of our spine and nervous system on a daily basis.

2. Being pain free is a lousy way to judge your health

While pain is a great motivator, most conditions begin long before you feel anything. Heart disease begins long before a heart attack, cholesterol builds long before any symptoms, and your cavity worsens long before the toothache. Only seven percent of the nervous system can detect pain. While back pain, spinal problems and nervous system dysfunction are common, that doesn't make them normal. They are common because it's also common that people don't take care of their spines and maintain their nervous system integrity. You'd never think of not going for a dental or eye exam; why on earth would you not get a spinal exam? Proper chiropractic care, proper spinal stabilization exercises and proper nutrition are essential over the course of your lifetime to optimize and maintain its function. After all, why would anyone want anything less?

3. Exercise is essential but it's not enough by itself

Isn't exercise enough to maintain my spine and nervous system? In a word, no! Exercise is one of the **5 Keys to Health,** but it can't replace the other four (proper nutrition, optimum nervous system function, adequate sleep and healthy beliefs). One of the greatest myths shared by people who think they are healthy is that exercise is all you need. In fact, exactly the opposite is true. Exercising on a misaligned spine or pinched nerve can actually create damage. Imagine driving your car more but on misaligned wheels. What will eventually happen? Recent medical research shows that degenerative changes in the spine begin within two weeks after even a minor spinal misalignment from everyday activities. Most of the world's top elite athletes likely exercise more than you ever will yet they all receive regular chiropractic care. Tiger Woods has been quoted as saying that his chiropractic care is as important as practicing his golf swing. Lance Armstrong takes his chiropractor on tour with him. Dan O'Brien, once dubbed the world's greatest athlete, states he couldn't have done it without chiropractic care. And don't forget MVP Hall of Famer Joe Montana's television segment on chiropractic to billions of people before the Super Bowl. If you don't have a chiropractor, what do these athletes know that you don't?

We have the knowledge to perform heart transplants, kidney transplants and liver transplants. The only nervous system transplant that I've ever heard of occurred on an episode of Star Trek where Worf (a Klingon) had such a procedure performed on him. He actually died during the operation but came back to life as apparently Klingons have a back-up nervous system. Humans do not. If you wish to have a lifetime of health you need to take care of your spine and nervous system.

Optimum Nervous System Function = Optimum Health

22

Can You Really Lose 23 Pounds in Thirty Days?

The answer may surprise you

There are few things in health that have more varying opinions than weight loss.

There are those who will settle for nothing less than washboard abs, others who are so obsessed that they are borderline anorexic and yet others who will put more effort into defending their right to be fat than making the effort to lose that fat.

When it comes to measuring your fat it could be determining your BMI, measuring your waist, obtaining your fat percentage or weighing yourself six times a day.

And when it comes to how to best lose that weight there are more programs than the amount of pounds that most people lose. And then gain back. And lose again. And gain back yet again.

Do we really need to lose fat?

In a word, yes. While it's possible that someone who is considered five to ten pounds overweight may be healthier than someone who is considered to be at an ideal weight, the truth is that most of the western world needs to lose fat and keep it off. According to the best research, if current trends continue, within twenty years eighty-six percent of the population will be either overweight or obese. This essentially means that out of every ten people almost nine of them will be overweight or obese.

Contrary to those who believe that they can be fit **and** fat, most of this excess weight is in the form of visceral fat. This is fat that surrounds and engulfs your vital organs, releases its own hormones with adverse effects, lowers your metabolism, increases inflammation and cannot be removed through liposuction. Needless to say it poses a significant health risk to your well being.

What about these fantastic weight loss claims? Isn't one to two pounds a week what most experts say you should achieve?

Human nature is such that we want everything and we want it now. We may have had a lifetime of bad nutritional habits and poor health choices yet we expect to correct all this in a month or so (and with minimal effort or further bad health choices).

We also find that if we need to lose twenty-five pounds that a week of effort and deprivation to only lose one or two pounds may simply seem like too much effort. So how do we overcome this conundrum?

To properly answer this question we need to analyze where this idea of one to two pounds of weight loss per week came from and who are these so-called experts?

This belief comes from what is known as the "calories in – calories out" theory where your weight is solely dependent on calorie intake vs. calorie expenditure. Exercise more than you eat and you're supposed to lose weight – do the reverse and you're supposed to gain weight. Combine this belief with the fact that a pound has 3500 calories. The "experts" assume it's reasonable to eat 500 less calories a day (times seven days in a week = 3500 calories) or burn an extra 500 calories a day in exercise (times seven days in a week = 3500 calories) and hence we have one to two pounds of weight loss a week. Anything more than this and the experts assume the excess must be water loss, muscle loss or unhealthy.

So what's wrong with this theory?

Unfortunately these experts include most medical doctors, most dieticians and most personal trainers – and it's just plain wrong. I discuss this in detail and give numerous examples in my book "Nutrition Insanity", but to be brief it's not the quantity of calories so much as it's the quality of calories. What do you think would result in greater weight gain – adding an extra 1000 calories a day of junk food or an extra 1100 calories a day of raw broccoli?

A philosophy of doing the right things

The truth is that there really is no set number of pounds that should be lost in a week as there are many different factors affecting your rate of fat loss (vs. weight loss) and different people will simply respond at different rates. Therefore, instead of trying to achieve some pre-determined subjective number, simply ask yourself "are you doing all the right things?" This may sound almost too overly simplistic but in fact it is the best way to be successful in all your health endeavours. If you are truly doing all the right things either you will achieve your best results safely at whatever rate or at the very least you will know that you are doing all the right things.

So what about these 23 pounds in thirty days?

If you attempt to lose this much weight the wrong way (muscle loss, starvation, chemicals, unhealthy practices, high costs) then of course this is not appropriate. However, let me share a personal experience with you. My patients will tell you that I have always practiced what I preach but anyone can sometimes be distracted from an optimal level of health. As such, less than two weeks ago I just finished thirty days of following my own twenty steps in "Nutrition Insanity" to the letter, and I lost 23 pounds. It gets even better. Needless to say this was done in a very healthy way. It was also done eating real food and eating often. There were no potions or powders other than what I consider to be the best vitamin supplement (which everyone should take on a daily basis anyway) and the best protein powder in my post workout smoothie (which again should be taken by everyone). Now for the best part. Of those 23 pounds, 22.57 pounds were fat loss! So much for those so-called experts.

Now if I could market and guarantee this I would easily be a multi-millionaire if not billionaire but I'm not selling you any program costing thousands of dollars – I don't have one. Rather I have a book that retails for less than $20 and a common sense philosophy of doing the right thing. What you will achieve is the maximum that's right and healthy for you.

And then?

Obviously doing the right things doesn't end at thirty days. If you want to be healthy for the rest of your life you need to do healthy things for the rest of your life. But the beauty of my twenty steps is that it's easy to continue to follow and by doing so you'll achieve what most people don't – you'll lose the fat and keep it off at whatever rate is best for you.

*(It is now another thirty days since my original thirty day program and all 23 pounds are still off.)

23

Moving a Ton of Snow

How to safely shovel snow
without injuring your spine

Do you remember when you were a kid and you would look outside and say "boy did we ever get a ton of snow"? Well it turns out that you were being far more literal than you thought. If you consider that the average shovel full of wet snow easily weighs ten pounds and that a driveway could easily be two hundred shovels, you have two thousand pounds or one ton. It's no wonder then that each year so many people injure themselves on what many consider a routine activity. Imagine if you had to move two thousand pounds of bricks or firewood (in frigid weather I might add) without any warm up or with poor technique.

The injuries I see in my office go far beyond back pain. They also include shoulder problems, neck pain, hip problems and muscle spasm as well as a variety of injuries from those who slip or fall on the ice while shovelling. They also include those who re-aggravate old injuries or exacerbate unknown underlying conditions especially if you have a sedentary lifestyle. To help prevent injury, all of the following are recommended.

Prior to going outside

1. **Plan and assess** – If it's a large, wet snowfall get help or plan to break it up in segments. Is there supposed to be freezing rain tomorrow or will it be so warm that the snow will melt? If you have a heart condition, remember that a clean driveway is never worth dying for.
2. **Warm up** - You wouldn't (or shouldn't) do any other activity involving two thousand pounds without warming up and stretching.
3. **Choose proper attire** – This includes not only layering but also proper treads on your boots to prevent falls.
4. **Have the proper tools** – Shovelling snow and chopping ice require different tools. Ergonomic shovels may be useful provided you use them properly. Just like lifting weights, good equipment will never make up for poor technique.

Good technique

1. **Push.** It is far easier to push a ton of snow than it is to lift a ton of snow. When doing so be sure to keep your spine straight and push with your legs. Lift only when necessary.

2. **The three keys to lifting** – Shovelling snow is like lifting anything else.

   a) **Bend your knees** while keeping your spine upright.

   b) **Keep the load close to your body** (forgetting this defeats the benefits of bending the knees).

   c) **Remember that your feet do move.** Turn your feet, don't twist. There is no better way to injure your spine than to load it and twist it as this compresses the spine and puts significant pressure on the spinal nerves and discs. Repeated compression to this area is also likely to result in early degeneration. Use smaller loads when possible (just like lower weights and higher reps in a gym).

Prevention

True prevention goes far beyond good technique. Someone whose spine is in proper alignment and who has good core strength (these are two separate issues and each one is essential) will obviously withstand the rigors of snow shovelling and avoid injury far better than someone who has poor spinal alignment or someone who has never maintained their spine. Proper spinal alignment is also essential for proper nervous system function.

1. **Get a spinal exam** – It is amazing how everyone understands that they should have regular dental and eye exams yet they have never had a spinal exam. It should therefore come as no surprise that eighty percent of the population suffers back pain at some point in their lives. Chiropractors are doctors who specialize in the spine and nervous system and can detect and correct any underlying spinal misalignment long before you may feel anything.

2. **Should an injury occur seek professional help** – Again, chiropractors are your best bet as most injuries involve spinal joints and nerves as the underlying cause with the muscles then reacting. Be careful not to mistake the symptom of muscle spasm as the sole problem. Sharp pain, numbness or inflammation is rarely just a muscle problem. Simple muscle fatigue may also be benefited by massage therapy.

3. **Develop good core strength**. – This will also reduce the risk of injury but must be paired with proper spinal

alignment for optimum function as many of the best athletes in the world will tell you. Attempting to strengthen vertebrae in a misaligned position may actually lead to injury.

Snow shovelling can actually be an enjoyable form of winter activity and exercise provided the above precautions are adhered to. Should it be a rather excessive snowfall don't forget that a cool down period will also be of benefit. For more information please contact your family chiropractor or visit us at www.excellenceinhealth.com.

24

What Requires More Effort...
Your Health or Climbing
Mount Everest?

The answer to the above seems obvious to most – but it also speaks volumes on your views towards health.

On the one hand your health should come easy and natural whereas climbing Mount Everest is an incredible feat that requires great fitness, superior dedication, unwavering motivation and years of training. On the other hand, there is really nothing that you should be more dedicated and motivated about than your health. As opposed to years of training, your health should last a lifetime and without your health the above question would be a moot point as the feat of climbing Everest could never be achieved.

As such, the question really becomes why is it that some people are willing to go to incredible efforts to climb Mount Everest while others won't do anything to better their own health even though their life depends on it?

Don't let anyone ever tell you differently – you're the person most responsible for your health. Not me, not your MD, not the government and not your insurance company. You make the decision – I just want it to be an informed decision.

Good health is not a right that you're entitled to; rather it's your obligation that you achieve and maintain it over the course of your lifetime. It requires effort on a daily basis.

How much effort?

A little over four thousand people have successfully reached the peak of Mount Everest at over 29,000 feet since Sir Edmund Hillary and Tenzing Norgay first achieved it in 1953. Given the population of the world, this isn't a one in a million feat but rather it's closer to one in two million.

As if being one in two million isn't enough to stand out, in my opinion there are four Everest climbers who stand out even more.

Jordan Romero is the youngest climber to reach the peak of Everest at the age of thirteen. At the opposite end of the spectrum is Min Bahadur Sherchan, the oldest individual to reach the top, who achieved it just twenty-five days short of his seventy-seventh birthday.

Even more incredible is Tom Whittaker who reached the peak even though he only has one leg. Finally, there is Erik Weihenmayer, the only blind man to climb to the peak of Mount Everest.

What's your excuse?

If you've read my first full book, "Healthy Beliefs – Deadly Choices", you know I'm not a big fan of excuses. They're just an explanation (to yourself) as to why you did or didn't do something. For every person who has an excuse, there's someone else accomplishing their goal that chose not to make the same excuse.

Yes, it will never be my place to judge your excuses. And yes again, there might be the rare emergency that could be a valid reason, but guess what? Your body doesn't care what the reason is, it just knows something was or wasn't done. Think of the excuses the oldest or youngest Everest climber could have used let alone the excuse of missing a leg or being blind.

"Good health is not a right that you're entitled to; rather it's your obligation that you achieve and maintain it over the course of your lifetime."

What it really comes down to is how much you truly value your health and what effort you're willing to make to achieve it. You might never climb Everest but you can certainly begin making small steps on a daily basis to achieve better health. Even 29,000 feet began with the first step.

"To know and not do is not to know "

Confucius

Walk your talk and get your actions to be congruent with your supposed beliefs (assuming they are healthy beliefs). After all, if a blind man can achieve climbing Everest, you can certainly achieve better health.

About Dr. John Zielonka

Dr. Zielonka is one of Ottawa's best known health and wellness experts. His unique approach enables people to make informed choices and take an active role in their health. Only by looking at all the factors related to one's health can they maximize their true health potential.

Dr. Zielonka is a Doctor of Chiropractic, holds a Bachelor of Science degree in chemistry, is a certified rehabilitation doctor, a certified occupational health consultant and is the Director of Health and Wellness Canada. He is the author of "Nutrition Insanity", "Healthy Beliefs Deadly Choices" and co-author of the "World's Best Kept Health Secret Revealed, Volume 3" which pre-sold over 70,000 copies. His latest book, "Healthellaneous" hit bookstores in late November 2010. He is a lecturer and nutritionist and has made numerous television and radio appearances including spearheading the movement for National Health Day in Canada. He is the owner of the Ottawa Chiropractic & Natural Health Centre in Canada's capital, considered by many to be the premier centre for health in Ottawa.

His patients have included everyone from the world's fastest man, gold medal Olympic athletes, NHL, NFL and CFL players to past prime ministers, major corporations and being in the delivery room for newborn babies.

Dr. Zielonka, along with his wife Katherine, super-healthy daughter Breana, energy filled twin boys Tyler and Ryan, dog Jack and cats Haley and Dexter, strive to make the world a healthier place.

Dr. Zielonka's websites and other websites recommended by him:

www.drzonline.com

www.excellenceinhealth.com

www.corescience.ca

www.yourhealthstore.ca

www.healthybeliefs.ca

www.nutritioninsanity.com

www.healthbychoice.ca

Other books by Dr. Zielonka

Nutrition Insanity
A Serious Look at Nutrition…and our lack of it.
2009

Healthy Beliefs Deadly Choices
2008

The World's Best Kept Health Secret Revealed Vol. 3
2006

Dr. Zielonka's books are available at www.drzonline.com
as well as Amazon and all fine retail outlets.

They are also available at his health centre in the
World Exchange Plaza in downtown Ottawa, Canada.

Healthy Beliefs

Deadly Choices

How Your Beliefs Are Killing You

Dr. John Zielonka

What People Are Saying About "Healthy Beliefs Deadly Choices"

"Thank you for your timely book. I loved it! (Read it twice). Our society needs to be reminded that our health and well being are in our own hands. Even more – it's the beliefs we have about it which makes a difference. I choose to believe that my body is capable of healing itself as long as I give it proper nutrition, enough sleep, regular exercise and keep positive! That's why it was such a treat to read your "Healthy Beliefs, Deadly Choices". Those who are going to follow your advice will enjoy a healthy and happy life, abundance of energy and overall joy. Hope many more readers will decide to be responsible for their health! Looking forward to many more of your books!"

R. Zitikiene, Carleton University

"In his book, "Healthy Beliefs, Deadly Choices", Dr. Zielonka brings to light the many discrepancies in our so called "health care" system, and makes us really look at how we take care of ourselves, not only as individuals, but as a society. Dr. Zielonka makes it perfectly clear that we must first take responsibility for our own health, first and foremost, by thinking clearly about what our choices are and then acting on what makes sense."

Dr. Astrid Trim, President,
Momentum Healing Arts

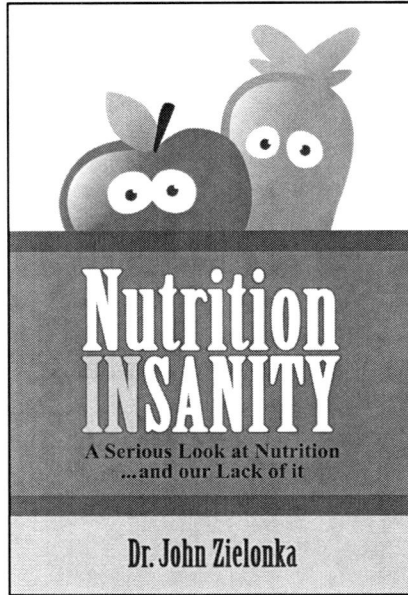

Nutrition INSANITY

A Serious Look at Nutrition
...and our Lack of it

Dr. John Zielonka

"**Nutrition Insanity** brings a little common sense to the often perplexing and myth filled world of nutritional health. As health care practitioners we are frequently questioned by our patients about whether the latest fad diet or miracle exercise program will work to help "lose weight". Dr. Zielonka's latest book provides clear, concise and well researched insights that not only break weight loss myths, but more importantly, provide straightforward answers to questions of eating for Health. This book is written in no nonsense language that will be appreciated by patients and practitioners alike. From osteoarthritis to cardiovascular disease, Dr. Zielonka provides simple strategies that will help you regain control over your body and make you feel and look great!"

Dr. Robert Fera B.Sc., H.K., D.C.
Integrated Wellness Concepts

#1 Best Seller

The World's Best Kept

Health Secret

REVEALED

VOLUME III

Dr. John Zielonka

and Leading Wellness Doctors

Book 3 of the Best Selling
Health Secret Series